The Hunt for the Parathyroids

T0256586

The illustrations on the cover are taken from Bernhard Siegfried Albinus' splendid anatomical atlas *Tabulae sceleti et corporis humani* (London 1749). The artist Jan Wandelaar made the skeleton as if it was alive and the idyllic frame with the grazing rhinoceros Clara and the park-like landscape connects science and the arts in a way that was typical of the 1700s zeitgeist.

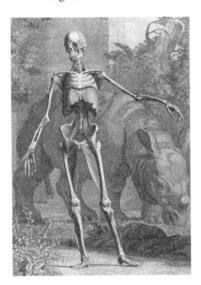
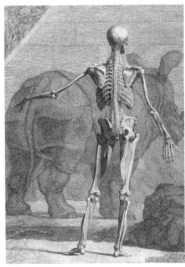

The Hunt for the Parathyroids

Jörgen Nordenström

Professor of Surgery
Karolinska Institute
Stockholm, Sweden

WILEY-BLACKWELL

A John Wiley & Sons, Ltd., Publication

Originally published in Swedish under the title *Körteljakten*, Karolinska Institutet University Press.

This edition first published 2013 © John Wiley & Sons, Ltd.

Blackwell Publishing was acquired by John Wiley & Sons in February 2007. Blackwell's publishing program has been merged with Wiley's global Scientific, Technical and Medical business to form Wiley-Blackwell.

Registered Office
John Wiley & Sons, Ltd, The Atrium, Southern Gate, Chichester, West Sussex, PO19 8SQ, UK

Editorial Offices
9600 Garsington Road, Oxford, OX4 2DQ, UK
The Atrium, Southern Gate, Chichester, West Sussex, PO19 8SQ, UK
111 River Street, Hoboken, NJ 07030-5774, USA

For details of our global editorial offices, for customer services and for information about how to apply for permission to reuse the copyright material in this book please see our website at www.wiley.com/wiley-blackwell

The right of the author to be identified as the author of this work has been asserted in accordance with the UK Copyright, Designs and Patents Act 1988.

All rights reserved. No part of this publication may be reproduced, stored in a retrieval system, or transmitted, in any form or by any means, electronic, mechanical, photocopying, recording or otherwise, except as permitted by the UK Copyright, Designs and Patents Act 1988, without the prior permission of the publisher.

Designations used by companies to distinguish their products are often claimed as trademarks. All brand names and product names used in this book are trade names, service marks, trademarks or registered trademarks of their respective owners. The publisher is not associated with any product or vendor mentioned in this book. This publication is designed to provide accurate and authoritative information in regard to the subject matter covered. It is sold on the understanding that the publisher is not engaged in rendering professional services. If professional advice or other expert assistance is required, the services of a competent professional should be sought.

The contents of this work are intended to further general scientific research, understanding, and discussion only and are not intended and should not be relied upon as recommending or promoting a specific method, diagnosis, or treatment by physicians for any particular patient. The publisher and the author make no representations or warranties with respect to the accuracy or completeness of the contents of this work and specifically disclaim all warranties, including without limitation any implied warranties of fitness for a particular purpose. In view of ongoing research, equipment modifications, changes in governmental regulations, and the constant flow of information relating to the use of medicines, equipment, and devices, the reader is urged to review and evaluate the information provided in the package insert or instructions for each medicine, equipment, or device for, among other things, any changes in the instructions or indication of usage and for added warnings and precautions. Readers should consult with a specialist where appropriate. The fact that an organisation or Website is referred to in this work as a citation and/or a potential source of further information does not mean that the author or the publisher endorses the information the organisation or Website may provide or recommendations it may make. Further, readers should be aware that Internet Websites listed in this work may have changed or disappeared between when this work was written and when it is read. No warranty may be created or extended by any promotional statements for this work. Neither the publisher nor the author shall be liable for any damages arising herefrom.

Library of Congress Cataloging-in-Publication Data

Nordenstrom, Jorgen.
  [Korteljakten. English]
  The hunt for the parathyroids / Jörgen Nordenström. – 1st ed.
    p. ; cm.
  Originally published: Stockholm : Karolinska Institutet University Press, c2009.
  Includes bibliographical references and index.
  ISBN 978-1-118-29969-2 (pbk. : alk. paper)
  I. Title.
  [DNLM: 1. Endocrinology–history. 2. Parathyroid Glands. 3. History, 19th Century.
4. History, 20th Century. 5. Parathyroid Diseases. WK 11.1]
  616.4–dc23
                                                   2012032886

A catalogue record for this book is available from the British Library.

Wiley also publishes its books in a variety of electronic formats. Some content that appears in print may not be available in electronic books.

Cover image: © Lars Paulsrud
Cover design by Andy Meaden

Set in 9.5/12pt Minion by SPi Publisher Services, Pondicherry, India

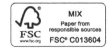

MIX
Paper from
responsible sources
FSC® C013604

1   2013

Contents

Preface

Relatively few people are familiar with the tiny vital organ composed of four small glands known as the parathyroid glands, and even fewer know the fascinating story behind their discovery, function, and diseases. Yet parathyroid disorders are not unusual; they comprise the third most common hormone-related illnesses after diabetes and thyroid disease.

When I as a young surgeon more than 25 years ago cautiously began operating on patients with enlarged parathyroid glands (hyperparathyroidism), I felt a mixture of keen enthusiasm and subdued anxiety. Equipped with rudimentary surgical skills, we young surgeons were allowed to assist our older colleagues on a few cases, eventually undertaking our first operations – this was the way the craft had been taught from time immemorial. For patients with hyperparathyroidism, we could try operating on our own after having assisted on 4–5 cases. We were instructed that if the diseased gland had not been found within two hours, a more experienced colleague would step in, usually locating the sought-after gland within minutes in the carefully exposed area of the neck.

In the early 1980s, the disease was shrouded in mystery, somewhat the way it still is today. We had heard stories about patients who had been locked up on psychiatric wards and who had later been completely cured after undergoing an operation, or patients who had been operated on unsuccessfully a number of times. The actual surgical procedure ranged from being easy to perform to being almost impossible. Hormone analysis at that time was unreliable, patients were hospitalised for 3–4 days, given a standardised low-calcium diet and their urine collected over 24-hour periods for an analysis of its calcium concentration. In some places patients were in intensive care units for days after their operations due to the risk of cramps.

The situation today is entirely different with better diagnostic options, more precise blood analyses, the possibility of using isotopes and ultrasound to confirm an enlarged gland prior to operation, and post-operative hospital stays usually no longer than one day. However, the mystery and challenge of the disease still remains: not every patient with hyperparathyroidism has elevated calcium or hormone levels, the localisation procedures are not entirely reliable, the operation is not always successful and a few patients actually do not have the parathyroid disease that we assumed they had prior to operation.

When a patient is referred for an opinion as to whether an operation should be performed, there are usually only two items of information: elevated calcium and hormone levels. Before surgeons meet a patient, it is impossible to know whether they are going to see someone with clear symptoms and complications caused by the illness, or who has no complaints at all, appearing no sicker than the surgeon. When I meet patients with hyperparathyroidism, I make a point of asking them what they know about this illness. I often find that they have fragmentary or almost non-existent knowledge of the disease. Using pencil and paper, I explain the cause of the illness to the patient; describe where the glands are normally found, what the effects of the disease might be and how the operation will be performed. In 15 minutes I relate the story behind the disease – a condensed version of the story that is told in this book. While I sit drawing and discussing with my patient, the spirits of long-gone colleagues and researchers who contributed to our knowledge of the disease hover over us. These include Ivar Sandström (who first described the organ), Fuller Albright (who described the mechanisms of the disease), Felix Mandl (who performed the first operation), and many others. The patients Albert Jahne and Charles Martell are also there – the first patients to be diagnosed with hyperparathyroidism. The expression "standing on the shoulders of giants" that Google Scholar uses as its motto seems especially appropriate here; today's surgeons and physicians are able to see a little bit farther ahead as a result of our predecessors' discoveries.

This book is intended for both informed readers with an interest in medicine and science as well as people with a particular interest in the subject. Naturally, an account aimed at such a broad audience causes problems for the individual reader; some may find the text to be too medically detailed, while others may feel that the simplifications that have been made do not fully describe the oftentimes complex processes and mechanisms that are associated with the hormone and its target organs.

Certain sources have been particularly important in terms of background material. Fuller Albright's posthumously published book, *Uncharted Seas* (1990), has been a model and a source of inspiration. A number of decisive articles (see the Reference List) have related different parts of the history of the parathyroids in condensed form and contributed valuable information. However, the most important source of information has been the Internet, in particular the books that have been scanned and collected in the Google

Book Project that have made it possible to find information about researchers, their research, and events that otherwise would be almost impossible to find.

Librarians at a number of libraries, especially the Karolinska University Hospital Library, the Karolinska Institutet University Library, Hagströmer Medico-Historical Library, the Carolina Library at Uppsala University, the Owen Wangensteen Historical Library at the University of Minnesota and the Institute for Medical History at the University of Vienna have been of great assistance in helping me acquire articles. Additionally, material from the Nobel Archives was kindly provided by the Nobel Committee for Physiology or Medicine.

Last but not least, I would like to express my thanks to my friends and colleagues who have read through this manuscript correcting errors and mistakes and otherwise improving the content. Special thanks to: Paul J. Rosch, John MacFie, Philip K. Petersen, S. James Adelstein, Isaac Austin, Helen Kearney, Dan Traub, Rowan Stephenson and Oliver O'Sullivan. Financial support for the printing of this book has been provided by the Maj and Lennart Lindgren Foundation and the Åke Wiberg Foundation.

As a practicing endocrine surgeon who has cared for patients with parathyroid disorders (both prior to and sometimes after operations), it has been both an educational and pleasant challenge to try to chart the history of this remarkable organ and the countless researchers and doctors who have contributed to our present understanding of its function and the treatment of its diseases.

Jörgen Nordenström
Stockholm, 2012

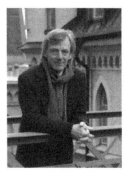

Introduction

This is the story of a tiny organ that normally does not weigh much more than 100 mg and was completely unknown some 100 years ago. These small glands, hidden away among the fine structures in the neck, had remained undiscovered for many centuries, partly because the organ is composed of four separate, minute, and visually nondescript structures, and partly because no one knew of any function or illness that could be associated with it. The introduction of thyroid operations made it very clear that this organ had a vital function. One of the pioneers of surgery, the American surgeon William Halsted, declared, "it seems hardly credible that the loss of bodies so tiny should be followed by a result so disastrous." The organ was given the name *parathyroidea* (parathyroid gland) and the small organ would later be found to secrete a chemical substance, a hormone. The discipline dealing with the effects of hormones would later come to be known as endocrinology.

The story began in 1877, when a young medical student made an anatomical discovery, and continues on to this day. The world has undergone extreme changes during this span of time. Today it is difficult to imagine how people lived at the time when the parathyroid gland was discovered: no electricity, telephone, radio, and of course no TV or Internet. The horse and carriage was the most important form of transportation; railroad networks were in their infancy, and cars and airplanes were still science fiction. Sailing ships or steamboats were the order of the day when a long journey was undertaken. Steam or sailing ships carried people on long journeys, but few had ever voyaged more than some 100 km away from home. Fewer still had visited other countries or other parts of the world. People lived and worked in the same neighbourhood.

Like many disciplines, medicine was not very developed. The possibilities of making a diagnosis or providing treatment were quite limited and most patients could hardly count on being cured. Most of the diseases that are well-defined today were not yet known, and some of the illnesses that could be found have either been eradicated or are now very rare. Hardly any of the medicines that were around then are still in use today, and surgery was only performed as a last resort when a patient's life was in danger.

The medical advances made during the last 100 years have occurred as either the result of ground-breaking discoveries or more often through gradual observations and incremental addition to the established knowledge base. A historical perspective is therefore an important component of the scientific process, and the researcher who wants to be successful should be a Janus figure – looking both forward and backward at the same time. There are those who maintain that truly original discoveries cannot be made, nor is it possible to understand the breakthroughs that have been made, without knowledge of history.

The science of medicine began to change at the end of the 19th century with the introduction of physiology (the study of "how things work"). With its physical/chemical and experimental methodology, physiology was a complement to descriptive anatomy ("what things look like"). Claude Bernard, the Father of Physiology, described his approach to the methodology of scientific research in his book, *Introduction á l'étude de la médecine expérimentale* (1865), laying down many principles that are still valid today. Bernard maintained that it was the experimental method that advanced science, and that this was built upon proving the correlation between cause and effect. The basis for this lies in the use of objective data to confirm or refute one's hypothesis, often with much repetition and investigation of competing theories. Bernard argued that the scientific search is a kind of yearning for the unknown, an aspiration that is never entirely satisfied, continually leading the researcher to carry out new experiments. According to Bernard, a true scientist searches for the truth, and although he may not find the entire truth, he will find fragments of the secrets of the universe, and it is these fragments that constitute science itself.

At the beginning of the last century, the research process was often described in terms of a journey: a physical journey as a metaphor for an intellectual one – an exploratory expedition to investigate the secrets of life instead of the geographical world. The last unknown frontiers of the great continents and the oceans were in the process of being charted and many of the world's highest mountains were being climbed. This new generation of researchers often saw themselves as the heirs of the historical adventurers and soulmates of the explorers of their own times. Like Odysseus, Christopher Columbus, David Livingstone and Fridtjof Nansen, they wanted to explore unknown territory, ever higher, deeper and farther away. Some would be successful, breaking new ground in the sciences.

Lewis Carroll published the hilarious tale, *The Hunting of the Snark* (1876), ten years after *Alice in Wonderland*. *The Hunting of the Snark* is the tale of an unlikely expedition that was undertaken by an implausible crew to find an inconceivable but valuable creature – a Snark. The crew members were not quite sure of what they were looking for and the actual search was a goal in itself. They also realised that if they ever were to find a Snark, it might not be quite what they had expected from the beginning, but rather something entirely different, maybe even something frightful – a Boojum.

> "He had bought a large map representing the sea,
> Without the least vestige of land:
> And the crew were much pleased when they found it to be
> A map they could all understand.
>
> 'What's the good of Mercator's North Poles and Equators,
> Tropics, Zones, and Meridian Lines?'
> So the Bellman would cry: and the crew would reply
> 'They are merely conventional signs!'"
>
> Lewis Carroll, *The Hunting of the Snark*, Fit the Second

Equipped with a nautical chart completely devoid of any land markings, they embarked on a journey with an uncertain end. At times they mixed up the bowsprit with the rudder, resulting in the ship sailing backwards for days, and when they thought they were sailing in a westward direction, they were actually sailing east.

The charting of the parathyroids, their function and diseases also began as an expedition with no map. A medical puzzle containing many pieces. Not only a Boojum – an illness was discovered, but also a Snark – and not just one but several. Some of the most prominent anatomists, pathologists, physiologists and biochemists, internists, and surgeons of the last two centuries would all come to contribute to an understanding of the function and diseases of this minute organ. The list includes names that are familiar to most medical doctors: Virchow, Kocher, Billroth, Ringer, Marie and Pierre Curie, Albright and Yalow. A number of them would have the good fortune of being invited to travel to Stockholm to receive the Nobel Prize. What these and other scientists succeeded in doing was to identify conditions that were related to parathyroid disorders, to describe the normal function of the gland, and to develop chemical techniques to determine the concentration in the blood of the hormone produced by the parathyroids. The tiny organ would be shown to play a crucial role in the body's regulation of calcium and, as time passed, it would be shown that calcium performed a vital function in human and animal physiology and biochemistry, as well as in different signaling systems at a cellular level. This would also result in a description of the complex interaction between the hormone and its target organs, the determination of the structure of the hormone, a charting of the receptors in the cells of the target organs, the confirmation of the signal paths and alterations in the gene expression and, most importantly of all, the discovery of effective treatment strategies for the illnesses caused by organ disorders.

In a broader perspective this medical-historical narrative is a historic exposé on the conditions and nature of humanity itself – the search for truth and purpose, the hopes for success and the pathetic failures, the groundbreaking discoveries that happened by chance, the missed opportunities, the struggles for fame and glory, the shattered illusions, and the lack of recognition. Yet most of all, this is a story about how successful research can contribute to promotion of health and curing of disease in patients.

A very long journey for a very small organ.

Chapter 1 **Sandström's discovery**

The story of the small glands that no one knew existed began in Uppsala, Sweden in the summer of 1877. Ivar Sandström was studying medicine at the university in Uppsala and was employed as a temporary research assistant to Professor Edward Clason in the Anatomy Department. Born in 1852, Ivar Sandström was the fifth child in a family of seven siblings. His father had died of cholera before the young Ivar had begun school, leaving behind substantial debts. Sandström began his medical studies in the fall of 1872 but it took a long time before he was able to finish. For economic, social and personal reasons, Sandström would not receive his medical degree until after 15 years of study. At that time, medical studies were usually completed in ten years. Sandström worked while he studied whenever he was able. He needed the summer job at the Anatomy department and although the salary was not very high, the money was useful.

August Strindberg, one of Sweden's greatest writers, described the early summer atmosphere in Uppsala at that time in these words:

> "It was spring once again and the friends had gone their separate ways, some had gone off to recruitment meetings, others to jobs in the countryside, and still others had returned to seaside resorts: he was alone in the city and envisioned a dreadful summer ahead in Uppsala where the summers could be unbearable.
>
> One afternoon in May he had sat reading in Carolina Park, and was now walking up the Castle Hill to see a bit of the horizon. The landscape is not exactly beautiful, but it doesn't make one long for the countryside, rather it awakens the imagination to thoughts of the sea; and he could see a steamboat push its way ahead through the dreadful fallow fields because he was born near the coast and was

The Hunt for the Parathyroids, First Edition. Jörgen Nordenström.
© 2013 John Wiley & Sons, Ltd. Published 2013 by John Wiley & Sons, Ltd.

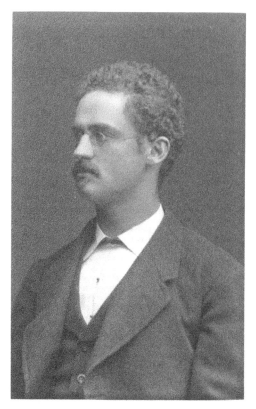

Figure 1.1 Ivar Sandström (1852–1889). Photo was taken when Sandström was about 25 years old at the time he made his unexpected discovery. (Reproduced from Uppsala University Library)

homesick. He envisioned all of the horrors of the coming summer and he wished it was autumn again."

Ivar Sandström was melancholy by nature, and perhaps he felt that way.

Sandström's introduction to medical research involved an event that must have been a shocking experience. It is a telling story about the state of the social-legal system and also perhaps about the level of medical knowledge in Sweden at the time. The scene was a place of execution in Central Sweden where professors Frithiof Holmgren, Axel Key and Edward Clason, along with Sandström and two other assistants from Uppsala had gone to make medical observations. What these medical men and over 2000 spectators were about to witness was the last act of one of the most renowned crimes in Swedish criminal history. Two relapsed criminals, Gustaf Hjert and Conrad

Tektor, had been sentenced to death by beheading for a double homicide two years earlier. The executions of Hjert and Tektor were scheduled to take place simultaneously on 18th May, 1876 at 7 am at two different locations; Hjert near the murder scene and Tektor on the island of Gotland. Clason and Sandström attended Hjert's execution with the intention to seize the opportunity to access fresh material for anatomical and histological studies. This was possible because Swedish law at the time considered the body of an individual who had been sentenced to death to be the property of the state. Professor Holmgren and his assistants were there to make observations in order to clarify "how long does a person maintain consciousness after the head has been parted from the body?"

Hjert's execution was a disastrous event. The authorities had urged locals to attend and even school classes with children were present. Immediately after Hjert had been beheaded, Professor Holmgren rushed to the head and looked into the eyes of the executed man. Holmgren found the eyes to be wide open with the pupils strongly contracted, but after 15 seconds the eyes were one-third concealed by the eyelids and the pupils began to widen. The face was without expression during the first minute after which some rhythmic movements appeared. "He is still alive!" one of the spectators shouted. After two minutes the face was still. While Holmgren made his observations several spectators rushed toward the body and gathered blood in spoons and bowls since according to popular legend blood from a recently dead person could be used to treat "falling sickness" (epilepsy). Holmgren later stated in a report that his study showed that "a decapitated head is incapable of making any observations" and that no consciousness remains after decapitation. The execution must have given indelible memories to the 24-year-old Sandström.

Sandström's job at the Anatomy Department was to dissect animals. It was slow and solitary work that required patience and precision. However, this did not worry him; being somewhat of a loner, he was most comfortable on his own. As in most of the anatomy departments around the world, comparative anatomy was a major subject studying the structural differences in anatomy between different animal species. It so happened that when Sandström was dissecting a dog he came across some structures that he did not recognise. In 1880 he wrote in the publication that would come to be the seminal text in the field:

> "Almost three years ago I found on the thyroid of a little dog a tiny growth, barely the size of a hemp seed which lay enclosed within the same capsule of tissues as that gland, though it was dissimilar in its lighter color."

He named the four small structures that he found in the neck *glandulae parathyroidea*:

> "An individual name for these structures seems appropriate . . . . both due to their substantial difference in appearance . . . . as well as their consistent localization."

The name *parathyroidea* was ingenious because it describes the exact location of the organ beside the thyroid (from the Greek *para*: 'beside' and *thyroidea*: 'thyroid gland').

It is understandable that this young medical student was initially skeptical as to whether he had really found an organ that had never been described before. Sandström wrote:

> "The existence of a hitherto unknown gland in animals that have so often been the object of anatomical examinations prompted a thorough search in the region around the thyroid in humans as well, even though the probability of finding something that had not been observed before seemed so minute that it was only out of consideration for the thoroughness of the examination, rather than in the hope of finding something new, that I undertook a careful investigation of the tissues surrounding the thyroid."

Obviously, neither Sandström nor his colleagues in the Anatomy Department could understand the potential significance of this discovery and further examinations were not undertaken for almost three years:

> "However, time and material did not allow for the completion of the examinations, and it was only during the winter that I had the possibility of continuing them."

After a hiatus of three years, Sandström continued with his project and carried out comparative anatomical studies on cats, oxen, horses, and rabbits, finding parathyroids in all of these animals. Naturally, the greatest challenge was to see whether parathyroids could be identified in humans. Here he was also very methodical, dissecting 50 corpses. He found that the structures were constant in 43 cases, but in five cases he found only one gland on each side, and in two cases only one gland on one side. Today we know that humans almost always have four parathyroids, and in exceptional cases one or a few more. Sandström discovered what every surgeon knows who operates on parathyroids nowadays, namely that the places where the four glands are located can vary and that it can sometimes be difficult to locate all of the glands. As an anatomist and histologist, Sandström could not go further than to describe the appearance of the organ. Naturally enough, he

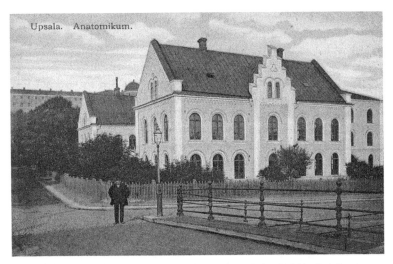

Upsala. Anatomikum.

Figure 1.2 The Department of Anatomy. Note the gas light showing that the photo was taken before electric streetlights were installed in Uppsala, at the time of Sandström's discovery.

had no clue as to what function, if any, the parathyroids had; however he assumed that they arose from undeveloped thyroid structures and predicted that "later on pathologists would find tumors in them."

It is probable that Sandström himself was very close to discovering a tumour in one of the glands he examined. He discovered a cyst (a clearly defined hollow space) in a gland. However, the slide material was so decomposed that he was not able to depict the microscope image in detail. The occurrence of cysts in normal parathyroids is unusual, but they appear occasionally in glands that have turned into tumours.

On reviewing the available literature, Sandström found that two researchers had observed the glands before him, although he "could not deny that there might have also been others." Sandström noted in his report that the two German pathologists, Robert Remak and Rudolph Virchow, had observed the parathyroids earlier. Yet these prominent pathologists had not understood that these small formations actually constituted an entirely unique organ, and that they had a particular function as well. Nevertheless, for some reason, the time was right for the parathyroids to be discovered. The pathologist D. A. Welsh stated in his dissertation in 1898 that some 20 German, French, Italian, and English researchers had observed the parathyroids during the years 1876–1881, around the time of Sandström's publication (1880), but none of these reports offered anything more than what Sandström had observed, and therefore they were largely ignored. Thus a number of anatomists had discovered the parathyroids independently around 1880 even though pathologists, and to some extent surgeons, had performed dissections in this region without having observed these minute structures.

Simultaneous (parallel) discoveries or inventions are, in fact, not that unusual. One of the more famous examples is the discovery of oxygen that was made by Carl Wilhelm Scheele in 1772 and by Joseph Priestly in 1774. That discoveries are made by several different researchers independently can often be explained by the fact that prior observations presented unexpected or conflicting results which caused people to begin questioning the existing concepts. A new discovery is in the air, so to speak, and this is usually a consequence of the intellectual climate or of new technical achievements at a specific point in time. The historian Robert Thurston describes the phenomenon of simultaneous discoveries in the following way:

> "Every great discovery is usually a compilation of a number of
> smaller discoveries or the last step in a development. It is not a matter
> of creation in the proper sense of the word, rather it is incremental
> growth. This is why the same discovery can often be made simultane-
> ously in different countries by different individuals. Often an
> important discovery happens before the world is ready to accept it
> and the unfortunate discoverer realizes that it is just as frustrating to
> be ahead of one's times as it is to be behind the times."

The reason why the parathyroids were discovered by several different scientists around 1880 was most probably related to the increased use of microscopes to describe normal and abnormally mutated cells and cell formations. The Dutch linen merchant Anton van Leeuwenhoek is credited with being the father of the microscope. He built a simple one-lensed microscope at the end of the 17th century and developed techniques for directing the light and improving the quality of lenses. In the mid-19th century, a microscope objective consisting of several weak lenses was developed and provided a sharper image and greater magnification by reducing the spherical aberrations (the chromatic effect) of light. The Zeiss optical company in Jena, Germany, developed mathematical formulas that offered the possibility of increased illumination, and the invention of the electric light further increased the technical potential. This development created the prerequisites for a new and previously unknown world – the world of microorganisms and cells. The German pathologists, especially Virchow, shifted the interest away from the organ to the cell.

Sandström had a great deal of experience with microscopic examinations, and for several years he was responsible for the microscopic laboratory exercises offered to the medical students. One of Sandström's colleagues in the

Anatomy Department, August Hammar, recalled that Sandström made his discovery during a microscopic examination of the thyroid of a dog. Thus it seems that he came upon the parathyroids via the microscope rather than on the dissecting table. The fact that electric light did not exist in Uppsala at the time of his discovery also suggests that Sandström did not initially see the gland during dissection – to be able to see a parathyroid gland *in situ* requires lighting that was hardly possible to achieve at that time. When Sandström realised that what he saw in the microscope was a new cellular structure he immediately ran to Professor Clason's room with his specimen. The professor was not there but Sandström caught sight of the microscope in the room. He was taken aback when he saw a slide with cells of similar appearance under Clason's microscope. At that instant, Clason appeared and Sandström wondered whether the professor had already seen what he wanted to show him. This was not the case, for Clason had in his microscope a slide specimen of cells from a pituitary gland – an organ which, with the deficiencies in histological staining techniques of those days, had a cellular structure very similar to that of the parathyroid gland. Today Sandström is most known as an anatomist; however his histological knowledge of the microscopic images of tissues and cells paved the way for his discovery. Sandström should therefore be considered outstanding both as a histologist and as an anatomist.

Sandström's discovery of the parathyroids was based upon the fact that he continued with studies on other animals and humans as a result of his first observations in dogs; and also that he systematically and carefully described both the microscopic image and the location of the glands and thus could establish that he had actually discovered a new organ. Even though others had observed the parathyroids before Sandström, they had not followed up on their observations nor had they understood that they were dealing with a novel organ. For this reason, Sandström has to be considered the person who discovered the parathyroids. Referring to Sandström's work, D. A. Welsh wrote:

> "I cannot too strongly emphasise the admirable precision and accuracy which characterise this earliest record of these glands in man."

While Sandström is arguably the first person to describe the parathyroids in humans, it turns out they had been observed earlier in a somewhat unlikely animal. In 1905, S.G. Shattock published a report which clarified that the parathyroids had in fact been observed prior to Sandström's discovery in the one-horned Indian rhinoceros *(Rhinoceros unicornis)*. Before 1830 there were only a very few single-horned Indian rhinoceros that had survived more than a few years in captivity. Clara was a spectacular exception. In 1738 this rhinoceros calf was captured when she was only a few months old after her mother had been killed by Indian hunters. Soon Clara was purchased by the Dutch sea captain Douwe Mout van der Meer who shipped the young rhinoceros to Holland. Clara became used to humans early on and she developed a taste for tobacco and beer, probably as a result of misdirected kindness on the part of the Dutch sailors. The creative van der Meer organised a travelling menagerie where Clara was transported around Europe on an enormous cart pulled by eight horses. The project was an economic success and Clara was on exhibition for over seventeen years in many different places throughout central Europe, admired by both ordinary people and high society including Frederick the Great and Louis XV. Clara became the source of inspiration for poems and musical compositions, and was immortalised in paintings, copper engravings, and on medallions and porcelain. Clara was a true celebrity. Jan Wandelaar, who illustrated Bernard Siegfried Albinus' monumental anatomical atlas (1747), was given a free hand to choose the background motif and he portrayed Clara on several pages grazing in a park-like landscape in order to make the anatomical drawings more attractive.

The English anatomist and zoologist Sir Richard Owen had convinced the Zoological Society of London to purchase an Indian rhinoceros in 1834 for the considerable sum of 1000 guineas (approximately €60 000 today). The rhinoceros had been a huge attraction at the zoo for 15 years when it died after breaking a rib and injuring a lung in a fight with an elephant. It was reported that the rhinoceros coughed up oxygenated blood – a sure sign of a lung injury. Owen was given the opportunity to dissect the cadaver. It must have been a gigantic project to dissect the cadaver of the rhinoceros that

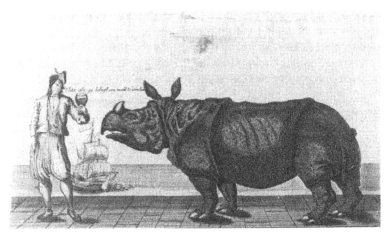

Figure 1.3 The Indian rhinoceros Clara being offered a glass of wine. Illustration on a poster, around 1748. (From L.C. Rookmaaker, 1998. Reproduced with permission, Kugler Publications, Amsterdam)

weighed almost 2 tons. Owen noted in a report on the dissection that the stench from the continually rotting cadaver did not exactly make the work any easier. In any event, he found a small, compact yellow structure in the expected location in the neck of the rhinoceros. In all probability, this was the very first observation of a parathyroid gland.

"Publish or perish" is the advice given to all young researchers by their mentors. Reporting scientific discoveries constitutes the foundation of an academic career. Research that has not been published has no value. Sandström knew this and he therefore sent his report to the local medical association's periodical, *Upsala Läkareförenings Förhandlingar*. This rather obscure publication contained announcements from the meetings of the medical association, debate articles and congratulatory speeches, abstracts from international journals, and case reports, as well as original medical findings. The publication's local character and readership is evident from the fact that it even published charts of the weather in Uppsala.

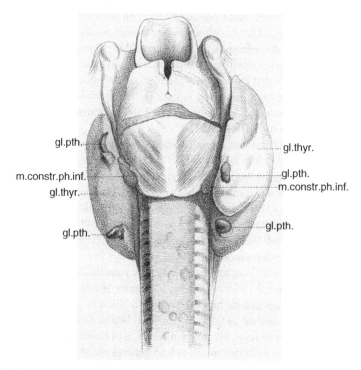

Figure 1.4 The parathyroid glands. Four parathyroid glands are depicted (gl.pth.) on the back of the thyroid. Drawing from Sandström's publication in *Upsala Läkareförenings Förhandlingar, 1880.*

In order to attract international attention, however, the work had to be published in a leading foreign periodical. Sandström therefore translated his Swedish manuscript into German and sent it to the doyen of pathology, Rudolf Virchow, for possible publication in his influential journal, *Virchows Archiv für Anatomie und Physiologie*. Publication in Virchow's *Archiv* would have surely attracted immediate attention in the worldwide research community. Surprisingly, and to Sandström's great disappointment, Virchow refused the piece. Sandström was urged to shorten the manuscript.

Indeed the manuscript was long, and it would have required some 30 pages of space in Virchow's periodical. However, the length of the manuscript may not have been the only reason it was refused. Many other articles published in Virchow's *Archiv* at the time were just as long, if not longer, and they dealt with topics that seem to be much less original or interesting to us today, such as "The Formation of Pseudo-cartilage in the Achilles' Tendon" or "Tuberculosis of the Liver." No, there were probably other reasons for the refusal. Some 15 years earlier Virchow himself had reported that he had found some small, round pea-sized lumps on both sides of the thyroid that "seemed to be neither lymph nodes nor formations stemming from the thyroid tissue" – a description that can correspond to parathyroid glands. It is remarkable that such a careful pathologist as he could have overlooked these constant structures that are routinely found in the region of the neck. Most probably, Virchow could not bring himself to let Sandström receive all the credit for the discovery of a new organ that Virchow himself had observed but had not pursued studying in detail.

Virchow's major scientific contribution was establishing the central significance of the cell in health and in sickness. This had influenced the entire development of medicine and had advanced pathological anatomy as an important instrument in clinical medicine. He was often described as strict by those who worked with him and he had absolutely no doubts about his own importance. As early as 1868 he wrote: "When they speak of The German School, they are speaking about me," a statement that paved the way for Virchow's position later on as "Germany's Pope of Medicine." He was known to be unwilling to acknowledge the contributions of others for discoveries that were at variance with his cell theory or that could in any way be linked to findings that he himself had made. Virchow gave no credence to the relation established by Ignáz Semmelweis between cadaveric contamination and puerperal fever. He was also skeptical of Robert Koch's work on tuberculosis and to bacteriological work in general, maintaining "anything that couldn't be seen with a dry lens wasn't worth looking for." When it came to the theory of cell development, his German colleague Robert Remak and the English researcher John Goodsir had articulated similar thoughts and thereby had laid the groundwork for Virchow's theory. What Virchow did, however, was to further develop the theory and make it better known to the world. The medical historian Erwin Ackerknecht maintained that Virchow's main contribution was that he gave the theory of cell development a deeper meaning and that he, tirelessly and with almost morbid energy, advanced his thesis in a way that no one had ever done before. The English pathologist Robb-Smith presented a similar opinion in an article published in *The Lancet* in connection with the centennial celebration of the publication of Virchow's *Cellularpathologie*:

> "It would certainly be rude to question the contributions of a great man during a jubilee; however, one must be aware of the fact that Virchow's contribution was not that he was the first to express the importance of the continual development of the cell, rather his major contribution was that he, with his propagandist skills, was able to convince his colleagues that his theories were the only ones that were correct."

It is perhaps against this background that Virchow's refusal of Sandström's work should be seen. Observations made by a medical student from Uppsala could not be allowed to indirectly point out an oversight that had been made by the "Pope of Medicine" in Germany.

All researchers have been urged to revise and abridge their manuscripts by editors of medical journals – 'kill your darlings' – Sandström, however, felt offended and he refused. He was neither the first nor the last person to have important discoveries rejected by editors of medical journals. Another example is Rosalyn Yalow, who had a report rejected that would later lead to the development of the highly sensitive radioimmunoassay (RIA), the method for measuring tiny quantities of hormones and other substances that would later result in her receiving the Nobel Prize. Australian doctors Barry Marshall and Robin Warren had an article rejected by the *New England Journal of Medicine* in which they demonstrated that stomach ulcers were caused by local bacterial infection with *Helicobacter pylori*, one of the last century's most sensational discoveries. They were also awarded the Nobel Prize.

Sandström made a huge mistake by not trying to get his article published in some other international periodical. His discovery was nevertheless noted as abstracts in three German medical yearbooks. One of these abstracts was written by Gustaf Retzius, a professor of Histology at the Karolinska Institute. Retzius was a person who truly supported Sandström and who helped bring attention to his discovery. Retzius, who was very influential and well-known internationally, was a member of the Royal Swedish Academy of Sciences and was on the committee that later gave Sandström a scientific award – the Florman Prize.

Today's scientists have an easier time when it comes to reporting new medical discoveries. The Internet has made all newly published information immediately available, and it is becoming more routine for scientific reports to no longer be printed as hard copy editions, but only to be published electronically. Google, PubMed, and other databases have resulted in the accessibility via individual computers to a volume of printed materials far exceeding those amassed in the world's libraries. The magnitude of accessible information today is almost incalculable. Google, which is surprisingly good for medical queries, contains references to more than 25 billion web addresses and more that 170 million searches are made in this database every day. Several years ago, Larry Page, who co-founded Google together with Sergey Brin, described Google's search capacity by saying that it could search through a 100 km high stack of standard size pages with tightly written information in less than half a second. Today Google can search through a 2000 km high stack of paper in the same amount of time.

Over the last few years a virtual global library has been in the process of being created, with Google aiming to scan all of the books ever printed and to collect them in an enormous database. Thus an old dream is being realised: the possibility of being able to store all printed knowledge and make it accessible to everyone in the world. The same dream lay behind the creation of the library in Alexandria around 300 BC, where an attempt was made to collect all of the papyrus scrolls that existed in the known world. It has been calculated that the Alexandrian library contained approximately half a million papyrus scrolls comprising about one third to one half of all of the written documents existing at that time. Yet even before the library was destroyed, the point had been passed where it would have been possible to contain all of the world's written documents in one and the same place. Since then, the constantly expanding mass of printed information has far exceeded the physical capacity to store it as printed matter. The universal library has been an unrealisable dream – up to now. Google's book project involves thousands of books being sent by truck from a number of libraries (including Stanford, Harvard, University of Michigan, Oxford and the New York Public Library) and then being scanned, page by page, in Google's special scanners. It has been calculated that there are 30 million printed books that it will take ten years to digitise. The goal is to make every printed page in every printed book in every language, searchable and downloadable.

Let us return to Uppsala. One might wonder why the regular staff in Sandström's department were not more supportive about emphasising the importance of making his findings known to a broader and, more importantly, international audience. In all probability, Sandström was not particularly receptive to such advice; he wanted to have things his own way. Another peculiar fact was that this young medical student stood as the sole author of such a comprehensive and thorough piece of work. At that time it was customary that more senior researchers almost automatically had their names inserted as co-authors of the works written in their departments. Today there are ethical rules for publishing that seek to regulate this, but at that time having a professor's name in the author list often conferred a scholarly legitimacy to the work. Another mistake Sandström made was to publish his findings as a research report and not as a doctoral dissertation. Had a doctorial thesis been published, Professor Clason, who was Sandström's mentor, would have had less difficulty in arranging an academic position at the university, something that he had eagerly tried to do. Sandström met with no success when he attempted to get the paper accepted as a doctoral dissertation after the fact.

Sandström was invited to give a lecture on his observations at the meeting of the Scandinavian Society of Natural Science in Stockholm in 1880. In a letter to his sister Anna he wrote that he was disillusioned because so few of the participants cared enough to come and listen to him, and the only person who had a kind word for him was a German professor who had not even been present when he spoke. Overall, he felt that the meeting was a farce because the delegates attending the gathering were busier trying to promote their own accomplishments than showing an interest in scientific questions.

At the Uppsala Medical Association's annual meeting on 17th September 1880 the usual keynote address was delivered, association business was discussed, and then the winners of the Large and the Small Hwasser Awards were to be announced. The jury panel for the Hwasser Awards had proposed that the first candidate for the smaller award be laboratory assistant Magnus Blix for his dissertation, "Ophthalmological Studies" with Ivar Sandström as the first runner-up for his paper, "On a New Gland in Humans and Several Mammals;" and Ivar Brandberg as the second runner-up for his thesis, "The Approximate Determination of Albumin in Urine." For the larger award, the jury panel had ranked Magnus Blix first, Ivar Sandström second and Count Karl Mörner third for his paper, "The Compounds of Alkali Albumin with Alkaline Soil and Copper." In spite of a lengthy discussion, a consensus could not be reached on who was to receive the awards, so the assembly had to take a vote. When the votes were counted, the Large Hwasser Award went to Sandström who received 250 Swedish *kronor* (approximately €1500 in today's currency).

*San*dström had every reason to be proud of his prize. His researcher colleagues, who competed with him for the award, would later become successful scientists and prominent representatives of academia. In just a few years Karl Mörner became professor of chemistry and pharmacology, and later, president of the Karolinska Institute. After the death of Alfred Nobel in 1896 a committee was formed to draw up the statutes for the Nobel Prizes.

Mörner was on that committee and was Chairman of the Nobel Committee for Physiology or Medicine from the time the first prize was awarded (1901) until his death in 1917. Magnus Blix was named Professor of Physiology at Lund University where he later became president.

In 1881 The Royal Swedish Academy of Sciences awarded the Florman Prize to Sandström. The minutes of the meeting of the seventh class (Medicine or Surgery) dated 5th March 1881, stated:

> "In connection with the announcement that the classes had been assembled to nominate a recipient of the Florman Prize, the secretary presented an account of the papers on the subjects of physiology and anatomy that had been submitted to the Academy during the past year, with particular note made of the fact that the Academy could reward works other than those that had been submitted to the Academy. After some deliberation, during which all of the members of the class agreed . . . that the findings published . . . in the Upsala Medical Association's periodical by the medical graduate Ivar Sandström were the most meritorious of all the papers presented that dealt with subjects eligible for the award, particularly in light of the significance of the discovery for normal as well as pathological anatomy and, additionally, for the accuracy of the examinations that had been performed by the author. The unanimous decision of the class is to recommend that the Academy award the Florman Prize to the medical graduate Sandström for the aforementioned work."

Sandström later collected the prize in the amount of 252 Swedish *kronor* and 12 *öre*, (again approximately €1500 today).

The article in *Upsala Läkareförenings Förhandlingar* would be Sandström's sole publication. He did not pursue his observations further, and for the rest of his life, he was plagued by mental illness and substance abuse. At times he suffered from heavy addictions to morphine, cocaine, paraldehyde and alcohol. In a referral in connection with his first hospitalisation for psychiatric care, Professor Clason stated that Sandström "had undergone treatment for morphine addiction many times." Sandström also had violent fits of rage with hallucinations; he had behaved threateningly and had attempted suicide several times. As time passed, he came to be seen as an increasingly tragic figure.

In the summer of 1886 Sandström was hospitalised at Uppsala Central Hospital due to insanity. The following was stated in his admission documents:

> "The patient was born on March 22, 1852 in Stockholm. He is married and has one child. No cases of mental or nervous afflictions are known in the family. He was taken in by a family of strangers when his father died, remaining in their care until he was 15 years

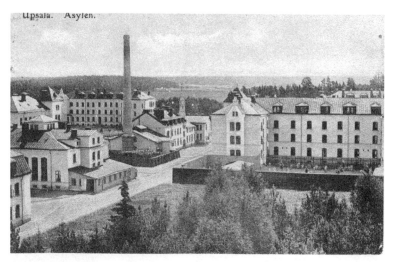

Figure 1.5 The asylum in Uppsala, where Sandström was an inmate due to insanity for various periods during the years 1886–1888.

old, at which time he returned to his home and his mother's care. He has always been of sound mind, has had a well-tempered disposition, lively and very sensitive, otherwise healthy except for recurrent bouts of gastritis. Has been sleep-deprived for a long time. He has been repeatedly treated for morphine use. His mood is volatile and agitated. His attention is impaired and his perception is not balanced. Has had visual hallucinations during the last weeks. His mental activity is normal. His speech is somewhat hesitant. His movements are slow and somewhat unsteady but are fully motivated. His pupils are either extremely contracted or dilated."

Date of Admittance: May 21, 1886
Diagnosis Upon Admittance: Acute Mania
Discharged: August 17, 1886. Recovered.

During the following two years, Sandström would periodically require psychiatric confinement for his psychosis. The concept of psychosis did not exist in psychiatry at that time; it was not until 1893 that Emil Kraepelin first classified psychoses into different illnesses: manic depression and dementia praecox (later called schizophrenia). Today's psychiatrists probably would have diagnosed Sandström as suffering from a manic depressive psychosis. This illness can now be treated successfully with lithium, of which one side effect is the development of enlarged parathyroids (hyperparathyroidism) and elevated levels of calcium in the blood. It is certainly an ironic twist of fate that if Sandström had lived today, he probably would have been treated

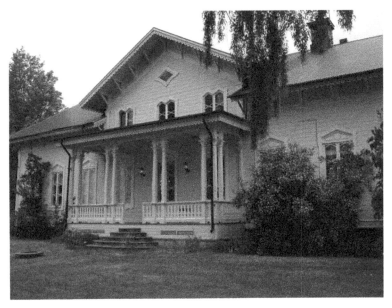

Figure 1.6 Askesta Mansion where Sandström spent his last days.

with lithium and he might have developed a disorder in the glands that he himself had discovered.

After an unsuccessful attempt to work as a medical doctor at a District Hospital near Uppsala, Sandström moved in with his brother Nils in Askesta, a small village in the northern provinces of Sweden. Nils was the foreman at the Askesta Sawmill which was one of the first and the largest steam powered sawmills in Sweden. The Askesta Mill was a booming business that generated enormous profits and allowed the entire region to flourish. It was in this dynamic and beautiful mill town setting that Sandström would spend his last years. Disillusioned, depressed, suffering from addiction and debt as well as having been abandoned by his wife Mary and their two young children, he found life harder and harder to bear. An announcement in the local newspaper, on 3rd June 1889, described his tragic end:

"An incident occurred yesterday at the Askesta Mill that will evoke sincere feelings of sadness and pain, not only among close relatives, but among comrades and friends as well. In a fit of insanity, Dr. Ivar Sandström MD, who had been visiting his brother Engineer Nils Sandström since February, took his own life by means of a revolver. Dr. Sandström had arisen early that morning, gotten dressed, and afterwards fired a revolver shot into his right temple in his bedroom. The bullet went through his head, exited through his left temple and lodged in the wall. This dreadful event occurred at about 6:30 am. The unfortunate man was found unconscious, but he showed weak vital signs throughout the day until his spirit gave up at 8:40 pm without ever regaining consciousness. Dr. Sandström was born on March 22, 1852. Naturally gifted, he soon made a name for himself as a result of his thorough and comprehensive studies, and early on he received several assignments as an academic teacher; accordingly, he was prosector as well as laboratory assistant and lecturer in histology at the university in Upsala. This all seemed to predict a promising future, when a debilitating nervous breakdown caused him to be afflicted with a mental disorder which broke the will of this gifted soul, and bouts of this illness finally caused his demise. He is survived by his widow, née Göransson (from the town of Gävle), together with two small children."

The day before this happened, Ivar was supposed to have said that it would have been nice if he had become a professor and had made a name for himself. He did not become a professor, nor did he ever come to experience the acknowledgement that he deserved for his research results. Yet the discovery of the parathyroids will always be associated with his name.

Sandström's discovery would turn out to be just the very beginning of the story of these small glands that had no known function.

Chapter 2 **Unexpected problems**

In a *Festschrift* published in commemoration of Rudolph Virchow's 70th birthday, the pathologist Friedrich von Recklinghausen described several patients who had an unusual skeletal disorder. One of the patients described in detail was Herr Bleich. He was 40 years old and a stonemason by profession. In April 1888 Herr Bleich had fallen three metres from a ladder and had landed on his left side. Eight days later he went to the hospital with pains in his left hip. It was assumed that he had a fracture and bed rest was prescribed. By August he was better and could walk with crutches, but two months later he fell again when he broke his collarbone. He was hospitalised once again and fractured his right femur while trying to use a bedpan. A physical examination a year later found him to be an emaciated patient suffering from intense skeletal pain. His upper arms, both his thighs and the lower parts of his legs were all crippled. His health deteriorated further and he died in October 1889.

Von Recklinghausen described a clinical picture where the calcium content of the skeleton was lower than normal and had been partially replaced by connective tissue and hollow cavities (cysts). He named the condition *osteitis fibrosa cystica*. In this condition the skeleton looks like Swiss cheese, and in advanced stages it is compressed, which leads to deformity and invalidity. In von Recklinghausen's description there was a notation about "a small reddish-brown lymph gland on the left side of the thyroid." Sandström's discovery made a decade earlier could have provided an important clue here if his findings had been known, because the description fits the complications related to a diseased enlarged parathyroid gland. The skeletal changes in *osteitis fibrosa cystica* are linked to one or several overactive and enlarged parathyroid glands and this clinical picture has been called 'von Recklinghausen's disease of the bone' ever since it was first described. Enlarged parathyroids as the underlying

The Hunt for the Parathyroids, First Edition. Jörgen Nordenström.
© 2013 John Wiley & Sons, Ltd. Published 2013 by John Wiley & Sons, Ltd.

cause was not understood until 1925 when the Austrian surgeon Felix Mandl operated on a patient with the same clinical appearance.

The remains of a 50-year old woman who lived more than 2000 years ago were found during archaeological excavations in the Dakhleh Oasis in Egypt. Examinations of her skeleton revealed a structure typical of *osteitis fibrosa cystica*, indicating parathyroid disorders have afflicted humanity for millennia.

There were several descriptions of isolated cases of parathyroid tumours some 20 years after Sandström's discovery. The first account by P. Santi (1900) was a case where the tumour was described as having been very large and having grown very rapidly "without having fulfilled the criteria for being a cancer." C. E. Benjamins (1902) described a case involving a parathyroid tumour that was "as large as a child's head," and he wrote in his report that "the case confirms Sandström's prophetic statement that tumours can probably be formed in the parathyroids." Whether this tumour really consisted of a diseased parathyroid gland seems dubious in retrospect, considering its exceptional size.

The appearance of skeletal disorders combined with enlarged parathyroids was first described by the German pathologist Max Askanazy in 1904. During the following years there were a great number of autopsy reports of patients with deformed skeletons and enlarged parathyroid glands. The first report of an enlarged parathyroid gland that was removed in an operation was provided by the Belgian surgeon C. Goris. At a meeting of the *Société Belge de Chirurgie* in 1905, Goris described how he had operated on a 22-year-old man who was found to have a cystic parathyroid tumour. It is evident from Goris' report that previous parathyroid operations must have been undertaken because he stated, "an enlarged parathyroid gland (or as he put it: a parathyroid goitre) is certainly not a rarity; however, it is not an ordinary tumour either." Another early operation was performed by the English surgeon Sir John Bland-Sutton who removed an enlarged ("the size of a pigeon's egg") parathyroid tumour sometime before 1911.

Yet the total picture was confusing, since a deformed skeleton could exist with or without signs of disease in the parathyroids, and enlarged parathyroids could appear without skeletal disease. In some cases there was an enlargement of all of the parathyroids while in other cases there was a benign enlarged tumour in only one of the glands. The underlying association was far from clear. If the changes in the skeleton were caused by a tumour, then one would expect that only one of the glands would have developed a tumour. On the other hand, if the skeletal changes stimulated a growth of parathyroid tissue, logically, all of the glands ought to be enlarged. Which was the chicken and which was the egg? Did the disease originate in the parathyroids or were the changes secondary to the skeletal disorder?

Surgery had made considerable advances by the end of the 19th century. There was mainly three factors that contributed to the advancement of surgery. Arguably, the most important of these were: the introduction of ether and later of laughing gas, which made it possible to perform painless operations; better hygiene and the adoption of principles for the prevention of infections (antiseptic and later aseptic procedures); and finally, improved techniques for controlling bleeding during operations. With no pain during operation surgeons did not have to operate as quickly as before. Over the ages, a surgeon's swiftness had always been synonymous with "skill." And that was no wonder: the shorter time the patient had to suffer during an operation, the better. It was said that Charles Darwin gave up his medical studies at the University of Edinburgh after he had witnessed an operation on a child that was performed without anaesthesia leaving him with haunting memories.

A vivid description of how an operation was performed in the mid-19th century can be found in Samuel Warren's collection of short stories, *Diary of a Late Physician* (1838):

"I had for several months been in constant attendance on a Mrs. St___, a young married lady of considerable family and fortune, who was the victim of that terrible scourge of the female sex, a cancer . . . .

A large Indian shawl was thrown over her shoulders, and she wore a white muslin dressing-gown. And was it this innocent and beautiful being who was doomed to writhe beneath the torture and disfigurement of the operating knife? My heart ached. A decanter of port wine and some glasses were placed on a small table near the window; she beckoned me towards it, and was going to speak.

'Allow me, my dear madam, to pour you a glass of wine', said I – or rather faltered.

'If it would do me good, doctor', she whispered. She barely touched the glass with her lips, and then handed one to me, saying, with assumed cheerfulness, 'Come, doctor, I see you need it as much as I do, after all . . . .'

At this moment, Sir___ approached us with a cheerful air, saying, 'Well, madam is your tête-à-tête finished? I want to get this little matter over, and give you permanent ease.' I do not think there ever lived a professional man who could speak with such an assuring air as Sir___!

'I am ready, Sir___. Are the servants sent out?' she inquired from one of the women present.

'Yes, madam,' she replied, in tears.

'Then I am prepared,' said she, and sat down in the chair that was placed for her. One of the attendants then removed the shawl from her shoulders, and Mrs. St___ herself, with perfect composure, assisted in displacing as much of her dress as was necessary . . . .

"At the instant of the first incision, her whole frame quivered with a convulsive shudder, and her cheeks became ashy pale. I prayed inwardly that she might faint, so that the earlier stage of the operation might be got over while she was in a state of insensibility. It was not the case, however, she moved not a limb, nor uttered more than an occasional sigh, during the whole of the protracted and painful operation . . . .

"Mrs. St___ recovered, though very slowly; and I attended her assiduously – sometimes two or three times a day, till she could be removed to the sea-side. I shall not easily forget an observation she made at the last visit I paid her. She was alluding, one morning, distantly and delicately, to the personal disfigurement she had suffered.

'But, doctor, my husband ___' said she suddenly, while a faint crimson mantled on her cheek – adding, falteringly, after a pause, 'I think St___ will love me yet!'

The situation had changed by the end of the 19th century. It was now possible to operate on organs that had previously been inaccessible for surgery. Extensive operations could be performed to surgically treat diseases that were previously incurable. A new world had opened up and the surgeons could try operating on organs and illnesses that had earlier been taboo: the liver, the brain, stomach ulcers, gallstones and abdominal tumours. During the same period of time explorers were investigating the interior of Africa, the surgeons were investigating the interior of the body. New operative procedures were described, new ground was broken and many advances were made. The surgeons became the new heroes of medicine. They had previously held a low status and it had taken a long time for them to become incorporated into the medical faculties. German-Austrian medicine was foremost in the world at that time, and the German-speaking surgeons were the most respected. Theodor Billroth in Vienna and Theodor Kocher in Bern were probably the most prominent of all.

At the end of the 1870s, Theodor Billroth felt that the time had come to resume thyroid operations. He had been a professor at one of Europe's most prestigious academic centres, the *Allgemeine Krankenhaus* in Vienna, for more than ten years. The hospital was an enormous building that was rather like an old square fortress with a park in the centre and could hold more than 2000 patients. It housed the world's largest maternity ward that went down in history as the place where Ignáz Semmelweis had identified the cause of puerperal or childbed fever 30 years earlier and tried to introduce antiseptic principles. Billroth's textbook, *Die allgemeine chirurgische Pathologie und Therapie in*

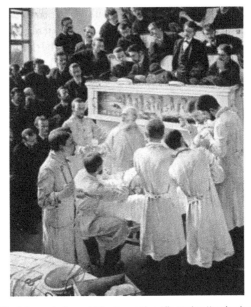

Figure 2.1 Billroth's surgical amphitheatre at the *Allgemeine Krankenhaus* in Vienna. Painting by Seligman, 1889. (Courtesy of Archive of Images, Department and Collections for History of Medicine, MedUni Vienna)

fünfzig Vorlesungen (1863), had given him a widespread recognition. His textbook was translated into ten different languages and republished in a total of 16 revised editions. This was the classic textbook of surgery at the time.

Billroth held a strong position on the faculty as well as in the world of European surgery, so he could do as he pleased without the risk of losing face or being criticised. At the *Allgemeine Krankenhaus* Billroth operated in an amphitheatre-like hall that had a railing around the operating table. The American surgeon George Crile described what happened during Billroth's operations:

> "Promptly at nine o'clock the wide doors of the clinic swung open, and Billroth, with his staff of twenty assistants, made a grand entrance. Everything was organized; each case had been studied. Billroth knew every detail. There was no more chance for an error than there was in the performance of a great play."

There were 200 seats in the operating theatre which were sold for ten *gulden* apiece. Inside the railing, guests of honour were seated in comfortable armchairs. Billroth was exceptionally knowledgeable, serious and innovative; yet the operations must have seemed like medical theatre.

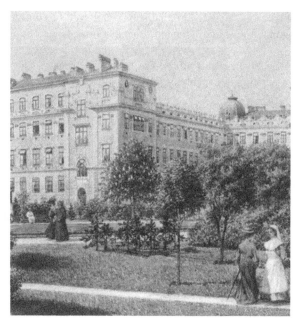

Figure 2.2 The Second Surgical Clinic at *Allgemeine Krankenhaus*. (Courtesy of Archive of Images, Department and Collections for History of Medicine, MedUni Vienna)

In many respects Billroth was a pioneer and was one of the first to keep statistics on the results of his operations. He carefully reported his results according to the number of deaths during the actual operations, the frequency of complications, and he even employed the concept of 5-year results which even today is used as a gauge of long-term results after different medical procedures. Billroth's awareness of potential problems with statistics is clear from his statement:

> "Statistics are like a woman; they can reflect the highest virtues and truths, but they can also be like a prostitute who can be used as desired."

Before Billroth moved to Vienna he had been a professor in Zurich where he had performed 59 thyroid operations, albeit with a mortality rate of 40%. Most of those that had died did so either due to infections or because of uncontrollable bleeding during the actual operation. These dismal results led Billroth to give up thyroid operations before he moved to Vienna. He was not alone in having abandoned the procedure. The *Académie Royale de Médicine* in France had simply forbidden thyroid operations in 1850. One surgeon stated that this was "a procedure that should not even be considered," and another felt that it was "one of the most thankless and dangerous procedures there is."

At the start of the past century, the American surgeon Charles Mayo described a situation that many surgeons recognised:

> "The surgery of the neck never seemed to enjoy the popularity of that of the abdomen, and goitre operations are not even today sought by the majority of surgeons. Those who were competent did not sufficiently often encourage operative relief until the absolute necessity rendered the mortality so high as to be almost prohibitive. The lay impression became such that operative measures were permitted only in the most advanced cases while semi-surgical, medical, mechanical, and electrical treatment flourished. In most cases, death came slowly and was looked upon as a relief from suffering, a result which satisfied everybody; but the death which follows operation is a shock to all and in but few instances is there a consideration of the fact that medical treatment had previously failed. Neither is the urgent necessity of the operation or the desperate condition of the patient taken into account, but the death has made a debit against the surgical side."

Theodor Kocher was the leading goitre surgeon during this era. He was technically skillful and very precise. He had conducted scientific studies in many areas that were relevant for goitre surgery: in blood coagulation and surgical haemostasis, iodine treatment and hormonal hypofunction after surgery (*cachexia strumipriva*). He received the first Nobel Prize ever awarded to a surgeon in 1909 for this work. He had also adopted aseptic techniques. Eventually, Kocher would be able to report excellent operative results for those times, with a mortality rate of 2%. The method for operating on the thyroid that he described is, to a great extent, still used today and the collar incision that is used is often called the "Kocher incision."

Theodor Billroth was the epitome of the new generation of academic surgeons: hard-working, daring, inventive and successful – a Christopher Columbus of surgery. He became somewhat of a cultural figure in Vienna – he was also an excellent pianist and a competent violinist who was very knowledgeable about music. His home was often the site of musical evenings, and Johannes Brahms dedicated his first two string quartets (Opus 51 in C minor and A minor) to Billroth. They were close friends, and Brahms often sought Billroth's advice and support when composing his pieces.

Billroth devised many new surgical procedures, perhaps the most famous of which were his types of gastrectomy. These operations involved removal of large parts of the stomach. They were frequently performed for patients with ulcers. Indeed, they continued to be carried out right up until the 1980s when the bacteria *Helicobacter pylori* was described in stomach ulcers. Proving the existence of these bacteria changed the treatment of the widespread disease of stomach ulcers from being a surgical procedure to being a treatment with antibiotics and proton pump inhibitors.

The situation for Billroth became untenable with the surgical department in Bern successfully performing goitre operations while his own department at the *Allgemeine Krankenhaus* in Vienna hardly operated on any goitre patients at all. This prompted Billroth to begin operating on thyroids again. From that point on, all of the goitre operations performed at Billroth's clinic were carefully documented in consecutive order.

One of Billroth's assistants, Anton Wölfler, described Case No. 11, a 35-year-old woman who had undergone a goitre operation in 1879, where an unusual course of events had developed. According to the description, it is apparent that the 45-minute long operation went well technically, but a number of different symptoms appeared on the day of the operation which "in all likelihood were related to the loss of the thyroid." A few hours after the operation the patient became restless, depressed and weak and urgently begged the doctors and nurses to help her because she felt worse than she had before the operation. It was observed that the area that had been operated on looked fine, there were no objective signs indicating a problem other than her symptoms, and that there was nothing more that needed to be done (*"nichts zu wünschen übrig liessen"*). The staff concluded that the patient was simulating. Several days later the patient's arms and legs started twitching, and at some point she lost consciousness. Gradually, the symptoms disappeared and the patient could be discharged. It was assumed that the symptoms were the result of an increased circulation of blood in the brain (cerebral hyperaemia), and having taken into account the fact that the patient had a uterus that was bent forward, it was determined that the combined picture probably indicated "hysteria." This was the first description of a new kind of complication as a result of the operation; however more cases would be described where the symptoms were more pronounced and the consequences more serious. The true reason for the patient's condition was not understood and it is interesting to note that the doctors, all of whom were men, tried to explain the symptoms with something that they obviously did not understand either: the female psyche.

Heidi, a 23-year-old Viennese seamstress, had been troubled by her large goitre for several years. It had made it increasingly difficult for her to swallow and she would get out of breath when exerting herself. An operation was performed in which her entire thyroid was removed. The operation itself was performed with no major problems, and the first days after the operation she generally felt quite well. On the third day after surgery, spastic twitching and muscle cramps appeared, causing her hands to remain in a position characterised as *der Hand des Geburtshelfers* (obstetrician's hand) since it is the same as the position taken for making a vaginal examination. She also had irregular twitching and pain on one side of her face during the following days and even more muscle cramps in her feet and legs. The cramps in her calves were so painful and she shrieked so loudly that it echoed throughout the entire ward. The pain increased even more the following days, sometimes with general cramps, several asthma-like attacks, muddled speech, and difficulty in swallowing. The situation became increasingly desperate with a very sick, frightened patient and distressed nurses who did not know what to do since the morphine and chloral hydrate they administered did not seem to have much effect. A high fever set in, the patient was bathing in her own sweat with increasingly worse cramping, and finally generalised muscle cramps and respiratory failure. Heidi was gone.

The surgeons were perplexed. No one could understand what had caused this new type of complication. The condition appeared to be similar to tetanus and was therefore called tetany. The condition came to be called *Schusterkrampf* (shoemaker's cramp) because of the similarities to the cramps caused by doing monotonous work using the muscles of the hand. Of the 38 thyroid operations that Billroth had performed, in ten cases the patients had tetany. It is somewhat ironic that Billroth, who had become so well-known for his many innovative surgical procedures, experienced a new kind of complication that made way for an entirely new field of research. No one could imagine then that these catastrophic complications would later come to be linked to the minute glands that Sandström was dissecting in Uppsala at the very same time.

The American surgeon William Halsted visited both Kocher and Billroth and observed their techniques during their thyroid operations. He noticed several differences. Kocher worked methodically and cautiously, carefully controlling the blood loss, while Billroth worked faster with less care of the surrounding structures and greater blood loss. He noted also that Kocher's patients seldom had cramps after the operation, while this was common for Billroth's patients. Kocher's technique, however, was not the only reason why his patients seldom had muscle cramps after thyroid operations. Kocher recommended that a small portion of the thyroid be left in place in order to avoid hypothyroidism, and he assumed (erroneously, as it would later be shown) that the remnant would prevent cramps. By leaving a small piece of the thyroid in place he probably avoided removing or injuring one or more of the parathyroids, thereby preventing hypofunction. It would take almost a half of a century, however, before the reasons for the terrifying complications of tetany could finally be explained.

One may ask how it was possible for 19th century surgeons to continue performing operations in which nearly half of the patients died of the actual procedure. Yet surgeons during the 19th century were not unique in introducing new surgical techniques that initially involved catastrophic consequences for some of the patients. The same thing happened during the mid-20th century as neurosurgery, transplant, and thoracic surgery evolved. During the 1950s, a relatively large number of kidney transplant operations were performed with kidneys from identical twins, usually with excellent results. However, using kidneys from deceased donors gave extremely poor results: in 1964 reports showed that out of 120 kidney transplant patients, only one patient's kidney was still functioning one year after the operation. The results were also discouraging for heart transplants. A compilation from 1971 showed that 146 out of 170 patients with heart transplants had died shortly after the operation. A telling conversation took place between the leading heart surgeons of the 1950s, John Kirklin and Walter Lillehai, when Kirklin expressed his frustration over so many patients dying after he had operated on them for a heart deformity in which all of the chambers of the heart were connected to each another. Lillehai answered, "Oh sure, that is a tough one, but we will learn to handle that too."

The regulations for the introduction of new procedures were drastically different then, but so were medical ethics. The surgeons, like everyone else, were frustrated that so many of their patients were incurably sick. When new technology was developed it was used first on the patients who were the sickest and who were considered incurable. They were going to die from their illness anyway. Thus patients were subjected to unproven methods, and many would pay a high price. The ethical reasoning was that the procedure could be motivated by the hopes of being able to use the method on future patients if the results could be improved. In this way some early patients paid dearly so that a much larger group of patients would hopefully be able to gain some future advantage. According to the ethical standards we hold today, it is unacceptable to expose individual patients to risk in order for future patients to be able to derive some benefit.

Jacob Erdheim was a professor of pathology in Vienna and he had a particular interest in pathological processes and experimental pathology. As a pathologist, he was quite aware of the problem of the fatal cramps that often occurred after the neck operations performed by Billroth and the other surgeons at the hospital. There were different theories for this, some people believed it was the loss of parathyroid tissue, others thought it was due to the removal of the thyroid and some believed it was a combination of the two. Erdheim realised that this debate could continue *ad infinitum* unless an experimental model was found to tackle the problem. What was needed was an animal model in which the parathyroids could be removed without injuring the thyroid. It so happened that rats had only one parathyroid gland on each side of the thyroid and they were just big enough to be seen with the naked eye. Using a red-hot needle, Erdheim was able to destroy ½, 1, 1½ or 2 parathyroids without injuring the thyroid. Some of the rats died, but many of them survived. The ones that survived had fairly mild cramps but they developed chronic parathyroid deficiencies. When Erdheim examined the animals after several weeks he found that their front teeth had become discoloured. The front teeth of rats are special in that they continue to grow throughout their entire lives. Erdheim was able to establish that calcium could only be deposited in the rats' growing teeth if enough parathyroid tissue had been left in the neck.

Erdheim also carried out the arduous task of performing a complete microscopic examination of the entire neck region of three patients who had died of tetany after undergoing thyroid operations, and he could not find any remains of parathyroid tissue in any of them. Having made these observations, he established that it was the responsibility of all surgeons to make sure that the parathyroids were left intact when performing thyroid operations so as to prevent the occurrence of cramps.

The connection between the parathyroids and bone loss was unclear for a long time. Erdheim maintained that pathological changes in the parathyroids were caused by skeletal disease and not vice versa. The objection to this was that usually there was only one gland that was enlarged, but this could be refuted by saying that the changes had to begin somewhere, after which all of the glands could gradually become affected. There were those who suspected that the tumours in the parathyroids could be the cause of von Recklinghausen's disease of bone (*osteitis fibrosa cystica*), but they were in the minority. Besides, how could an enlarged minute parathyroid gland weighing only a gram or two destroy an entire skeleton that weighed 2 kilograms? No, what Erdheim and the other leading pathologists maintained must be correct: the skeletal changes came first, with later enlargements of the parathyroids.

Erdheim showed with his experiments on rats that the function of the parathyroids could be maintained if they were transplanted somewhere else in the animal. The conclusion could thus be drawn that some kind of active substance was secreted into the bloodstream, and that the effect of this substance was not dependent on the glands being in their normal location. With these experiments, Erdheim was the first to show that the parathyroid gland was an organ that produced a hormone.

One of Billroth's surgeons, Anton von Eiselsberg, performed experiments on cats in 1892 where he transplanted half of the thyroid onto the wall of the abdomen and 5 days later removed the remaining half of the thyroid in the neck. Initially, the cats showed no visible symptoms, however when the

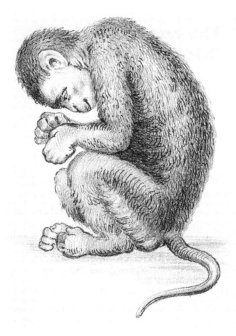

Figure 2.3 Muscle cramps in a monkey in which the thyroid and parathyroid glands had been removed. (A. von Eiselsberg , *Archiv f klin Chir,* 1895)

transplanted half of the gland was removed after several months, the animals quickly died from severe tetany. Even though Eiselsberg did not know the reason why the cramps began, he was the first to show that it was possible to transplant parathyroid glands and retain their function.

At the beginning of the 20th century, knowledge about the parathyroids extended no further than that the anatomical and microscopic characteristics had been clarified. The tetany that occurred after neck surgery happened when all, or almost all, of the parathyroids had been removed, but the exact reason for these cramps was unknown. The removal of all parathyroid tissue in animals resulted in the same type of cramps that could be observed in patients who had undergone neck operations. Hypofunction of the parathyroids affected the development of teeth in laboratory animals and somehow the skeletal changes in humans could also be linked to an altered function of the parathyroids, but the correlation was unclear. The transplantation of parathyroids within the same kind of animals could cure the tetany that arose from severe hypofunction; however, the results of transplants in humans were uncertain and temporary at best. Lastly, it had also been proven that the parathyroid gland produced a hormone.

Chapter 3 **The age of glorious discoveries**

The end of the 19th century was characterised by a pioneering spirit, a curiosity and optimism about the future in both Europe and North America. The birth of industrialism in the middle of the century had created new possibilities, significant achievements were made in all of the sciences, communications had developed, large segments of the population were on the move, and agrarian society began its gradual transformation into an industrial society. This was the Age of Glorious Discoveries. Alexander Graham Bell invented the telephone; Thomas Edison developed the incandescent light bulb and declared, "We will make electricity so cheap that only the rich will burn candles." Nicola Tesla invented alternating current; gasoline and diesel motors were developed, and it became possible to communicate via wireless telegraphy. The Wright Brothers made the first aerial flights and Henry Ford developed factories for the mass production of cars. All within the span of a few decades.

Central Europe was the motor of this expansion, and the World's Fair in Paris in 1899 was a magnificent manifestation of the ongoing technical revolution. The Eiffel Tower stood as the ultimate symbol of what could be accomplished by using the architecture and engineering techniques of a new era. Truly this was a complete turnabout compared to the previous century when the father of chemistry, Antoine Lavoisier, was sentenced to death by the Revolutionary Tribunal in Paris. When Lavoisier pleaded for a two week postponement of his own execution so that he could complete an experiment, the court judge, Jean-Baptiste Coffinhal, dismissed him with these words, "*La République n'a pas besoin de savants ni de chimistes*" (The Republic needs neither scholars nor chemists).

The period around the end of the 19th century and the beginning of the 20th century was also the era of exploratory expeditions. The interior

The Hunt for the Parathyroids, First Edition. Jörgen Nordenström.
© 2013 John Wiley & Sons, Ltd. Published 2013 by John Wiley & Sons, Ltd.

expanses of the major continents were being explored and explorers had reached both poles of the earth. Important archeological finds were made and there were major developments in the sciences. This entire epoch can be described as a massive expedition both at a macro and a micro level. Medicine, however, had not developed to the same extent as the natural sciences. The understanding of most illnesses was imperfect, and the possibilities of treating disease were very limited far into the 1900s. By and large, almost all of the drugs that were in use prior to the year 1900 were useless or ineffective, and those effects that could be observed were later attributed to the placebo ("sugar pill") effect. The emergence of methods for inducing anaesthesia and alleviating pain (William Morton, 1846), an understanding of the causes of infection (Louis Pasteur in the 1850s) and their prevention (Joseph Lister in the 1860s), X-rays (Wilhelm Röntgen 1895), and the discovery of blood types (Karl Landsteiner, 1901) were indeed major steps. Yet the real developments in medicine first gained momentum during the period between the two World Wars with the emergence of effective drugs such as thyroid hormones, insulin, sulphonamides and penicillin.

Many of the earliest pioneers in medicine were not doctors at all, but rather chemists or physicists. Louis Pasteur's discovery of bacteria and the vaccination technique is perhaps the most obvious example of a chemist launching a new medical discipline. Wilhelm Röntgen was a physicist, and his discovery of X-rays that could penetrate solid material immediately attracted a great deal of interest among both scientists and the general public. Suddenly it was possible to see structures inside the human body such as the skeleton without having to operate. Functional X-ray equipment was developed, and just a few years after the discovery of X-rays, there were radiology departments in many hospitals around the world. In comparison with countless other inventions, X-rays are one of the inventions that most rapidly found a practical medical application.

The French physicist Henri Becquerel was busy examining minerals that emitted radiation at the time when Röntgen made his discovery. Initially, Becquerel assumed that this radiation was a reflection of sunlight. After having stored minerals together with a photographic plate in a desk drawer, he found by chance that the plate had been exposed even in the absence of sunlight. He was then able to prove that uranium had the power to expose photographic plates and that this substance always, under all conditions, emitted radiation. Becquerel's observations signalled the beginning of one of the most fascinating and mythologised research projects in the history of science: the charting of the radioactive substances by Marie and Pierre Curie.

Marie Curie, who had moved to Paris from Poland only a few years earlier, began to systematically examine the ability of a large number of elements to

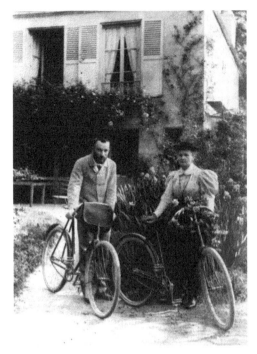

Figure 3.1 Pierre and Marie Curie with their newly purchased bikes shortly after their marriage in the summer of 1892. (Musée Curie, Paris)

emit radiation. She found that the metal thorium did so and she suggested the term radioactivity to describe the phenomenon. Marie examined the mineral collection at the *École de Physique* and she found a mineral fragment that emitted more radiation than could be explained by the amount of uranium and thorium that it contained. With her husband Pierre, who was already an established physicist, they together succeeded in discovering two new radioactive chemical elements. The first was given the name polonium after Marie's beloved homeland Poland, and the other radioactive element was named radium. Marie would later regret that the choice of names had not been reversed since radium became the more useful element in medicine.

For physicists, the Curies' discovery meant the stability of atoms had to be questioned. However, to be accepted as new elements, their atomic weights had to be determined. After many years of hard physical labor in a shed with a leaky roof in a Paris backyard, the couple succeeded in isolating one-tenth of one gram of radium chloride from several tons of pitchblende ore from the area of St. Joachimstahl in Bohemia, and they calculated the atomic weight to be 225 – a remarkable achievement that had been carried out under the worst possible physical conditions.

On 25th June 1903, Marie defended her thesis, *"Recherches sur les substances radioactives,"* at what must have been the most extraordinary dissertation examination in history. The candidate Marie was given the highest grade, and less than five months later she shared the Nobel Prize in Physics with her husband Pierre and Henri Becquerel. Two of the three members of her review committee (Henri Moissan in chemistry and Gabriel Lippman in physics), would also receive Nobel Prizes, though several years later.

In her book *Madame Curie – A Biography*, which is one of literary history's true bestsellers, Marie's younger daughter Ève described these rare radioactive elements in the following way:

"Radioactivity, generation of heat, production of helium gas and emanation, spontaneous self-destruction – how far we have travelled from the old theories on inert matter, or the immovable atom! Not more than five years before, scientists had believed our universe to be composed of defined substances, elements fixed forever. Now it was seen that with every second of passing time radium particles were expelling atoms of helium gas from themselves and were hurling them forth with enormous force. The residue of this tiny, terrifying explosion, which Marie was to call 'the cataclysms of atomic transformation,' was a gaseous atom of emanation which, itself, was transformed in its turn. Thus the radio elements formed strange and cruel families in which each member was created by the spontaneous transformation of the mother substance: radium was the "descendant" of uranium, polonium a descendant of radium. These bodies created at every instant, destroyed themselves according to the eternal laws: each radio element lost half its substance in a time which was always the same, which was to be called its half-life. To diminish itself by one half, uranium required several thousand million years, radium sixteen hundred years, the emanation of radium four days, and the 'descendants' of emanation only a few seconds. Motionless in appearance, matter contained births, collisions, murders and suicides. It contained dramas subjected to implacable fatality: it contained life and death."

Radium would later come to be used to treat cancer; however, careless use could also result in severe side effects. Initially, the Curies did not understand the risks involved in their work with radioactivity. Pierre often carried an ampoule of radium around in his pocket and Marie had radium beside her bed as a night light.

"When one works with studies using strong radioactive substances, one must observe special precautionary measures if one wish to perform precise experiments. The different objects that are used in a chemistry laboratory and that are used in physics experiments become radioactive very quickly. Dust particles, the air in the room, and clothes become radioactive. The air becomes conductive. In the laboratory where we work it has gone so far that we no longer have a single apparatus that is not contaminated by radiation."

Marie's admonition to carefulness primarily concerned the precision of the measurements and not her own physical safety. Even to this day, the Curies' laboratory books must be stored as hazardous materials, and anyone wishing to study them must follow special protective procedures – and this will continue to be the case for hundreds of years to come.

It was only later that the couple realised that radioactivity could be harmful to them. Perhaps the first signs of radiation sickness appeared as early as 1903. Marie and Pierre Curie were forced to decline the invitation to go Stockholm to receive their Nobel Prize. In a letter to the Royal Swedish Academy of Sciences on 19th November, Pierre after a polite introduction where he expressed their thanks for the prize wrote:

"It would be very difficult for us to travel to Sweden to take part in the festivities on December 10. At that point in time we can hardly leave Paris without causing disruptions in the teaching that has been entrusted to us here. Furthermore Mme. Curie was ill last summer and has not yet completely recuperated."

Several years later it was confirmed that Pierre suffered from muscle weakness and fatigue ("neurasthenia"), which in all likelihood contributed to the tragic accident that occurred in the spring of 1906 when Pierre was struck and killed by a horse and carriage as he was crossing a street in Paris.

Radioactively labelled substances would later become extremely important throughout the entire field of medicine as trace elements to describe the regulatory mechanisms of different substances and organs, to determine the composition of the body, to measure the levels of different hormones in the blood, and to visualise organs and pathological changes in certain organs when treating cancer and some other illnesses. Radioactivity would even come to have a decisive significance for the diagnosis of parathyroid disease.

Marie also made a great humanitarian contribution during World War I. She constructed mobile radiography units to make it possible to diagnose war injuries close to the frontlines. She begged to obtain vehicles which she

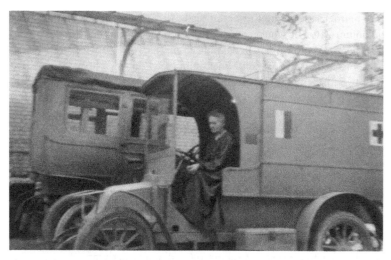

Figure 3.2 Marie Curie in her *"voiture radiologique"*. Photo taken during WWI. (Musée Curie, Paris)

then equipped with radiography apparatus that could be run on electricity generated by the ambulance motors. Twenty or so mobile units were fitted out with radiography equipment, and she kept one for herself which she used to travel around to the different battle sites. Marie had no background in either medicine or biology, but she taught herself anatomy from books she had brought with her and she did many of the X-ray examinations herself. She obtained a driver's licence so that she could drive her own *voiture radiologique* and started a teaching programme to train radiography nurses. In all, 150 *manipulatrices* completed a six-week programme after which they were assigned to radiography stations throughout all of France. She travelled untiringly, appropriating radiography equipment not needed at the hospitals and succeeded in creating 200 permanent radiography laboratories near the frontlines where thousands of radiographic examinations were done on soldiers wounded by bullets and shrapnel.

In time, Marie developed leukaemia and died in 1934 of aplastic anaemia. Perhaps the cause of her death was the radioactivity that she had been exposed to during her experiments, but it is more probable that she contracted leukaemia as a result of the radiographic examinations that she performed during World War I without any protection.

Death by radioactive exposure re-emerged over 70 years later with the lethal polonium poisoning in 2006 of the former Russian undercover agent Alexander Litvinenko, who was fatally poisoned in what was described as the first murder case where the victim died of acute radiation poisoning from polonium-210. The sequence of events was so spectacular that the story could have been taken from a fictional murder mystery or a spy story. Litvinenko was poisoned at the London Millennium Hotel during a breakfast meeting with two former colleagues from the Russian Military Counter Intelligence where polonium had been put into a teapot. Litvinenko fell ill the same day and died three weeks later. When polonium was discovered in Litvinenko's body, the police were able to find traces of radioactive polonium inside the teapot that was used at the meeting, on many of the hotel's dishes, as well as inside the airplane in which the two agents had flown. Polonium-210 is extremely poisonous if it is inhaled or swallowed, but the radioactivity cannot penetrate the skin if it is intact. Polonium is 250 000 times more poisonous than cyanide and a fatal dose for a human is about 50 millionths of a gram (50 nanograms). Polonium exits in very minute amounts in nature due to its short half-life (138 days) and is produced in nuclear reactors. The annual world production amounts to about 100 milligrams per year.

Chapter 4 **A gland in search of a function**

At the time of Sandström's death in 1889, the French physiologist Eugène Gley began to show interest in the small glands. Gley was trained as a scientist in French experimental medicine as it had been developed by Claude Bernard. An important discovery that had been made by Bernard was that the liver could store glucose in the form of glycogen which could be released as needed in order for the body to maintain relatively stable blood sugar levels between meals. The discovery that the liver could produce glucose became the starting point of Bernard's most famous contribution to physiology: the principle of the *"milieu intérieur"*. According to Bernard, a stable internal environment was a prerequisite for a free and independent life, regardless of variations in the intake of food and liquids, changes in temperature, etc. The parathyroids and their function of regulating the calcium concentration in the blood would come to play an important role in the entire complex system that regulates the internal environment.

Gley took on the task of studying the physiological importance of the small glands with great passion. Gley was initially more interested in the thyroid and he often used rabbits and dogs in his experiments. While working with rabbits, he found some interesting information in Krause's atlas of rabbit anatomy, *Die Anatomie des Kaninchens* from 1884. There Krause referred to Sandström's glands as they had been described in two German yearbooks and he even made reference to Sandström's article in Swedish published in *Upsala Läkareförenings Förhandlingar*. Through Krause, Gley became aware of the existence of the parathyroids and Sandström's discovery. He had referred to both Krause's anatomy book and to Sandström in one of his early publications. It is often stated that Gley re-discovered the parathyroids (that is, that he discovered the parathyroids without realising that they had already been identified earlier), however, this seems erroneous as he was aware of

The Hunt for the Parathyroids, First Edition. Jörgen Nordenström.
© 2013 John Wiley & Sons, Ltd. Published 2013 by John Wiley & Sons, Ltd.

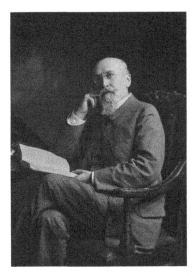

Figure 4.1 Eugène Gley (1857–1930), French physiologist. (Wellcome Library, London)

Sandström's discovery early on in his studies of animals. That Gley, who was strictly a physiologist, could have discovered and identified the parathyroids by himself without having been aware that they had been previously described, seems highly improbable.

In any event, Gley proved with his experiments that animals could sometimes have fatal cramps after thyroid operations and that this was associated with the loss of the small glands that he called the *glandules thyroidiennes*. Thus Gley became the first person to point out that the tiny glands had an important function, although his experiments were unable to rule out that the thyroid might have some role to play when tetany occurred.

Initially it seemed as though Gley was trying to create the impression that he himself should have priority for the discovery of the parathyroids. This was neither the first nor the last time (as would later be shown in connection with the discovery of insulin) that Gley claimed priority for discoveries that had been made by others. For many years he was the general secretary of *La Société de Biologie* and he reported on his research findings in over 15 abstracts in the periodical, *Comptes Rendus de la Société de Biologie*, which were based upon lectures that he had delivered at meetings of the Society during the period 1891–1895. Objective data were seldom presented in these reports; instead they were running texts of abstracts of the experiments that he had conducted.

Few researchers outside of France adopted the name *glandules thyroidiennes* which impelled Gley to propose the name "Sandström-Gley's glands" in 1896, but by that time Sandström's priority for the discovery had already been generally acknowledged. After Gley had been convinced that the thyroid and the small *glandules thyroidiennes* were separate organs with different functions, he began to use the term "parathyroid glands" – the name that Sandström had coined.

Gley's research became the starting point for intense interest in an organ that was obviously vital – at least in experimental animals – and it was in this way that Gley re-established Sandström as the researcher who should be granted priority for the discovery.

Experiments on animals in which the parathyroids and the thyroid were removed either separately or together were conducted by different researchers in order to elucidate the exact function of the parathyroids. It became apparent, however, that it was not all that easy to study parathyroid function in this manner. The results were often inconsistent and some researchers maintained "the operation is, with very few exceptions, more or less impossible." The problems they confronted were myriad: the parathyroids were difficult to identify accurately with the naked eye, the places where the glands were located varied between species as well as from one individual to another within the same species, the number of glands varied and they could be found among lymph glands, in the thymus, or be enclosed within the thyroid gland. To prove that the parathyroids had a function different from that of the thyroid was not easy, and many investigators doubted the actual significance of the parathyroids. One researcher commented upon the problem of trying to cause a parathyroid deficiency in animal experiments by saying that it was proof of the wisdom of nature: it was difficult to remove all of the parathyroid tissue since the organ had a vital function. For a long time, Gley had a rather diffuse conception of the anatomy and function of the parathyroids. As late as 1901 he maintained that there was some kind of physiological association between the thyroid and the parathyroids. He also thought (erroneously) that bulging eyes which could be seen in patients with thyreotoxicosis were caused by parathyroid dysfunction.

Like many others, Gley experienced difficulties with his interpretations because of his insufficient knowledge of the anatomical particulars of the parathyroids. He found that dogs usually died of tetany when their parathyroids were removed, while other animals were rarely affected in the same way. The explanation was that the location of the glands varied between the species and, in some animals (e.g. cats and rabbits), one of the two pairs of parathyroids was actually enclosed within the thyroid gland. Some animal species consequently had both an "inner" and an "outer" pair of parathyroid glands. Using this new information, the pathologist Guilio Vassale conducted animal experiments in which he could accurately remove either the thyroid or the parathyroids and was able to show conclusively that the fatal cramps were a result of parathyroid insufficiency and that the thyroid was not involved in the development of tetany. It was thus demonstrated that the thyroid and the parathyroids had two distinct functions: loss of the thyroid led to chronic problems including a lower metabolism, and loss of the parathyroids led to acute and often life-threatening symptoms.

Vassale was nominated for the 1905 Nobel Prize by three Italian professor colleagues. He advanced to a full evaluation, but in the end the prize was awarded to Robert Koch for his studies on tuberculosis. Perhaps it was just as well that Vassale was not awarded the prize as one of his theories regarding the parathyroids' primary function was that they were involved in the clearance of harmful substances from the body. The mistaken theory of an antitoxic function of the parathyroids lingered for a long time, and contributed to delaying the understanding of the parathyroids' true function of regulating the metabolism of calcium by some 20 years.

In time, Gley became a renowned professor of biology at the *Collège de France*. However, he came to be seen as an odd researcher, as illustrated by an event that occurred at a meeting of the *Société de Biologie* in December 1922. The major medical event at that time was the discovery of insulin by the Toronto group of Banting, Best, MacLeod and Collip. At the Paris meeting, Gley requested that an envelope that had been sealed back in 1905 be opened in the presence of the assembled delegates. The documents that had been deposited at the *Société de Biologie* described animal experiments from 1900–1901 in which Gley had blocked the pancreatic duct and collected an extract that could lower the blood sugar levels in dogs that had diabetes. In the main, this was the same method that Banting and Best had used to prove the existence of insulin; yet Gley maintained that he had made use of it 20 years earlier. He gave no explanation as to why he had not published his findings earlier instead of archiving them. The medical historian Michael Bliss has pointed out that it was unethical of Gley not to have published his results so that other researchers could build upon these potentially important findings. Gley realised too late that he had missed one of the most important discoveries in medicine. He congratulated MacLeod for having made "*une grande simplification*" of his method, an odd comment since no one had known about his experiments.

Documents in the Nobel Archives reveal that Gley was nominated for the Nobel Prize in 1921 for his studies on the function of the parathyroids. Eleven professors, all Gley's colleagues in France, had written individual letters in what must have been a coordinated campaign. The Nobel Committee was unsympathetic to the proposal, however, and Gley did not advance to the full evaluation process. It is possible that the announcement of his experiments with an extract from the pancreas a year later was an attempt to fuel the fire in hopes of a possible new nomination for the prize. An alternative explanation could be that he aspired to gain some part in the discovery of insulin. Frederick Banting and his collaborators in Toronto had managed to isolate insulin during the winter of 1921–22, a discovery that was generally expected to be awarded a Nobel Prize, which happened quite rightly in 1923. That Gley would get credit for the discovery of insulin and any part of this prize was of course out of the question. Instead, he is remembered as the researcher who discovered that the parathyroid gland has a unique physiological function.

There are many examples in the history of medicine where chance circumstances have led to epoch-making discoveries. Henri Becquerel's discovery of radioactivity is one of the many examples of this and we will see other examples later. What is presented less often are the cases where researchers have incorrectly interpreted or misunderstood the implications of their observations and have therefore missed making important discoveries. Gley's attempt to extract a substance from the pancreas that would lower blood sugar levels is an example of one such overlooked discovery. Another overlooked discovery was the antibacterial effects of sulphur. The German chemists at I. G. Farbenindustrie synthesised and patented sulphanilamide as early as 1909, but they had failed to observe the antibacterial properties of the substance. W. Jacobs and M. Heidelberger at the Rockefeller Institute were searching for antibacterial substances and synthesised the substance a second time in 1915, but they chose not to perform microbiological tests because they felt that sulphur was "too simple a substance." In 1935 the pharmaceutical company Bayer AG launched *Prontosil*, which was the first effective drug for treating infections. Sulphur had no effect on bacterial cultures: it only worked after it had been metabolised in the body. French chemists at the Pasteur Institute discovered later that the active substance was sulphanilamide. The use of sulphur during World War II saved the lives of many thousands of soldiers.

The problem of fatal muscle cramps was observed at all surgical departments that performed goitre operations, and Johns Hopkins, where William Halsted was a surgeon, was no exception. During the period 1878–1880, Halsted visited the leading surgery departments in Europe, including Vienna where he took part in some of the operations that Billroth conducted there. Halsted also did experimental studies on the physiology and surgical treatment of the thyroid in the surgical laboratory of the *Allgemeine Krankenhaus*. He became good friends with Anton Wölfler, one of Billroth's assistants, who was interested in the problems related to tetany that could occur after neck surgery. In this way Halsted took an early interest in the parathyroids and at the beginning of the 1900s he charted the blood supply of the parathyroids and experimented with parathyroid transplants. Halsted became very influential in the entire field of surgery, and he established standard procedures for breast cancer surgery, new methods for hernia operations, and introduced the use of rubber gloves during operative procedures. As a young surgeon, Halsted had experimented with cocaine as a local anaesthetic. He performed many experiments with cocaine on himself and, like Ivar Sandström, he came to suffer from an addiction to narcotics.

Coca leaves have been used since time immemorial by the Indians of South America. The Spanish settlers brought coca to Europe, but the practice of chewing coca did not become particularly widespread. The use of coca took a new turn when Albert Neiman succeeded in producing and chemically isolating the cocaine alkaloid in 1860. Cocaine then began to be used as both a stimulant and a pharmaceutical. In 1886 the pharmaceutical chemist John Pemberton created a drink using cocaine as one of the ingredients that was launched as a "drink for mental alertness." It was later named Coca-Cola. It was not until 1903 that cocaine was eliminated from Coca-Cola. Vin Mariani was another popular drink that contained cocaine. Sigmund Freud began using cocaine early on to treat his own depression as well as those of his patients. He became an ardent advocate of the use of cocaine for depression and as a treatment for morphine addiction. He also noted the anaesthetic properties of cocaine. During the latter half of the 19th century, the use of cocaine became common in both artistic and medical circles. When the risks of cocaine became known around 1900, the use of the drug was criminalised, after which its use diminished. Besides Freud, the list of doctors who used cocaine also included Arthur Conan Doyle. However, one of the individuals who suffered the most was Halsted. He tried to conceal his addiction in every possible way, and his colleagues at Johns Hopkins, including William Welch and William Osler, tried to help him overcome his addiction. One of Halsted's young surgeons, who would later make a name for himself, was Harvey Cushing. He had noted that, for no apparent reason, Halsted was not at the clinic on many occasions, that he was periodically confused, that he sometimes sweated profusely, and that his hands often trembled. The underlying reason for Halsted's behaviour never became apparent to Cushing or to most of his colleagues.

Even though experimental animal studies pointed clearly to a role of the parathyroids as the cause of tetany following surgery, there were still those who doubted their role as being solely responsible for the observed dramatic effects. Indeed it had been shown through experiments on the adrenal, thyroid and pituitary glands that endocrine organs had important functions; however, these organs were prominent and rather large. It did not seem plausible that a few glands the size of hemp seeds that could hardly be seen by the naked eye and that were located in different places in the neck region, could have any important function. Erdheim, who was convinced early on that the parathyroids had an important function, showed understanding toward those who doubted the facts: "The contrast between the minuteness of the parathyroids and the fatal effect of the removal of the organ is so immense that it is natural that many people are still skeptical."

Final proof that the parathyroids and the thyroid were two independent organs was left to nature itself. The Austrian internist Friedrich Pineles reported eight cases where the thyroid glands were missing due to a congenital anomaly in the foetus. Each of these cases had normal parathyroids. There has never been a case reported where the parathyroids were completely missing, which indirectly suggests that the loss of this organ is fatal. Even though the knowledge of the importance of the parathyroids had been framed by dramatic events, including fatalities, the underlying causes of tetany would not become apparent until the 1920s.

Chapter 5 **The calcium connection**

Calcium was discovered in 1808 by Sir Humphry Davy while working at the Royal Institution of Great Britain. Davy had developed a method based upon the discovery made by Alessandro Volta a few years earlier that electric current could be generated by alternately stacking zinc and silver plates and separating the two metals from each other with a wet cloth. Volta could not explain the phenomenon, but he observed that the electricity "was real and could be felt by the hand." Davy found that the electric current was not generated by the metals themselves, but rather that an electrochemical phenomenon occurred between the metals and the liquid. The insight that Volta's battery was a chemical process led Davy to develop a method, electrolysis, by which different elements can be isolated by sending an electric current through melted elements and solutions. Using electrolysis, Davy succeeded in isolating more chemical elements, including calcium, potassium, sodium, magnesium, strontium, and aluminum, than any scientist had done previously.

It was not until the beginning of the 1880s that Sidney Ringer, a researcher and doctor at University College Hospital in London, clarified the biological function that calcium had over and above its role in building up the skeleton. Ringer used isolated frog hearts to study the effect of different substances contained in blood on the heart's ability to contract. In one of his early publications he demonstrated that frog hearts placed in a solution of sodium and potassium chloride would contract normally for several hours. Shortly after Ringer published these findings he realised that a mistake had been made. The mistake was discovered by accident when Ringer's laboratory assistant Fiedler was on leave and Ringer himself made a saline solution. It turned out that it could not keep the heart contracting for more than a few minutes instead of the four hours that had been the case when the experiments had been done earlier. When Ringer confronted Fiedler with

The Hunt for the Parathyroids, First Edition. Jörgen Nordenström.
© 2013 John Wiley & Sons, Ltd. Published 2013 by John Wiley & Sons, Ltd.

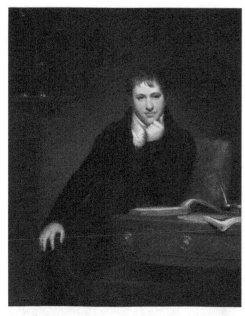

Figure 5.1 Sir Humphry Davy (1778–1829). (© National Portrait Gallery, London. NPG 4591 Sir Humphry Davy, Bt by Henry Howard oil on canvas, 1803)

the problem he found out that Fiedler had used tap water and not distilled water, as Ringer had assumed. When they analyzed the tap water it was shown to contain calcium in a concentration that was almost as high as the concentration usually found in the blood. In a series of experiments, Ringer was able to show that calcium was essential for the heart's ability to contract. Without calcium the heart soon stopped in a cramped state, "water rigour". Only when calcium was present in the solution could the chambers of the heart expand so that the heart worked normally.

In principle, Ringer's experiment had shown that calcium had hormone-like effects and worked like a kind of "first messenger" to trigger a physiological effect. After experimenting with a large number of solutions having different salt concentrations, Ringer was able to define the mixture of sodium, potassium, chlorides, bicarbonate and calcium that best and longest could maintain normal heart function in the frog. The recipe came to be known as "Ringer's solution." This solution, or variants of it, is still used today in biological laboratory experiments around the world and as an oral rehydration solution for patients suffering from, or at risk of, dehydration.

The significance of calcium in preventing cramps and maintaining normal muscle function was documented as early as 1883, at a time when

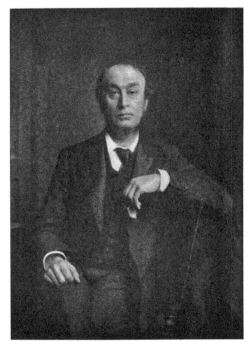

Figure 5.2 Sidney Ringer (1835–1910), English physician and physiologist. (Wellcome Library, London)

surgeons throughout Europe began observing the problem of cramps following neck surgery. In hindsight, it is difficult to understand why the leading clinicians and researchers at the universities in Vienna and Bern and at different institutions in London did not make the connection between low calcium levels in the blood and muscle cramps. Ringer published his findings in a number of articles during the period 1883–1890 in the periodical *The Journal of Physiology*, but apparently no one linked together the experimental and clinical observations that had been made in different locations. The connection between the parathyroids, muscle cramps and calcium would not become apparent until several decades later.

The German-American physiologist Jacques Loeb, like Ringer, was curious as how different salts affected physiological functions. Loeb also found that calcium was imperative to prevent muscle cramps and to sustain a number of other functions. His later research would be more focused on questions about the origins of life, and his spectacular findings would make him one of the most renowned scientists in the United States. Loeb spent his summers doing research at the Marine Biological Laboratory in Woods Hole on the southeastern coast of Massachusetts, using sea urchins, jellyfish and various other marine animals. He showed that by chemically changing the surrounding environment, an artificial fertilisation of sea urchin eggs could occur that resulted in their developing into normal larvae. In the same manner, frog eggs could develop normally through physical-chemical manipulation without ever having been sexually fertilised. Fatherless frogs originating from virgin births! The discovery provided the newspapers and the tabloids with new material for imaginative interpretation and fantasy. The headlines in the *Boston Herald* from 1899 illustrated this: "*CREATION OF LIFE. STARTLING DISCOVERY OF PROF. LOEB. LOWER ANIMALS PRODUCED BY CHEMICAL MEANS. PROCESS MAY APPLY TO HUMAN SPECIES. IMMACULATE CONCEPTION EXPLAINED. WONDERFUL EXPERIMENTS CONDUCTED AT WOODS HOLE.*"

The general public's thoughts about the consequences of the discovery seemed boundless. There was talk about maiden ladies giving up sea bathing on hearing of Loeb's discovery and there were women congratulating the scientists for "having finally freed the woman from the shameful bondage of needing a man to become a mother." There were even bizarre religious statements to the effect that "science of this recent day is entertaining as a possibility what Christian faith accepts as actual in the case of the most notable birth that ever occurred."

Loeb, a serious and hardworking researcher who had been used to keeping a low profile, had in a very short time, advanced to become a prominent scientist and a public figure. In media, he came to symbolise the brilliant scientist. Later he would also come to serve as the model for the researcher Max Gottlieb in Sinclair Lewis' *Arrowsmith*. In this novel, Lewis lets a country doctor misconstrue Loeb's findings:

> "Well, this fellow said Arrowsmith was always arguing with the preachers – he told some Reverend that everybody ought to read this immunologist Max Gottlieb, and this Jacques Loeb – you know – the fellow that, well, I don't recall just exactly what is was, but he claimed he could create living fishes out of chemicals."

Loeb had demonstrated that the mechanisms of heredity and cell division were separate processes. He maintained that biological life originated from physical chemistry, and that the art of biological engineering could be used to initiate all biological processes and even to create new varieties or species: artificial parthenogenesis in frogs and sea urchins were simply examples that confirmed this hypothesis. Loeb's research proved, among other things, that calcium and other substances could function as a "second messenger" inside the cells by being able to initiate a surge of biochemical events that could

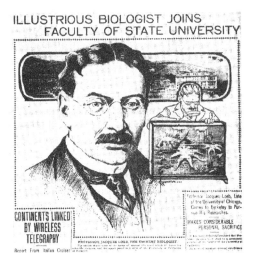

Figure 5.3 Jacques Loeb (1859–1924), German-American physiologist and biologist depicted on the front page of the San Francisco Examiner. (November 12, 1902) (By permission of Oxford University Press, Inc.)

trigger different physiological effects, for example a muscle contraction, the initiation of cell division, or the secretion of a hormone.

It had been established in the early 20th century that calcium was a vital ion for maintaining important physiological effects. It had, of course, been well-known for a long time that calcium was needed to provide support and stability in the body (the spine and the long bones in the arms and legs) and to protect important structures (the skull, the rib cage, and the pelvis). It had long been doubted, however, that calcium could have a general and fundamental significance for practically all cell systems. It was simply difficult to imagine that one of the body's most common ions could be one of the body's essential substances for maintaining physiological functions. It was not until the mid-1900s that it was understood that calcium had a great many important functions, both inside and outside the cells, such as for muscle contraction, nerve conduction, the coagulation of blood, and for numerous enzyme functions. The list of calcium's effects would later become even longer: calcium initiates new life at conception, it regulates parts of the development of the foetus, it controls the metabolism of a number of different substances, it regulates the transport of different materials through cell membranes and it affects our ability to learn and remember things. Indeed, it would later become clear that it is very difficult to find physiological functions in the human organism not dependent upon calcium.

An interesting question is why, amongst many other inorganic ions, has calcium achieved such a special status as a key messenger substance for a myriad of physiological functions? In comparison with other possible substances, calcium has a number of favourable properties which include its molecular structure, valence state, binding strength and ionisation potential. Calcium's role in biology is best understood from a perspective based on its intrinsic value as a divalent cation able to precipitate inorganic and organic anions rapidly. Paradoxically, the reason for this special status emanated from the necessity of primitive cells to control the calcium ion as it has a number of toxic properties. A high calcium ion concentration causes damage to intracellular organelle structures, aggregates proteins and nucleic acids and precipitates phosphates involved in energy transfers – events that would cause instant death of the cell.

The person who first put calcium on the agenda as far as the parathyroids were concerned was a young pathologist at Johns Hopkins, William MacCallum. His interest in the parathyroids had been roused by Halsted around 1905 and he performed a number of experiments where he gave parathyroid extract to dogs that had had their parathyroids removed. Some of Halsted's patients who were suffering from muscle cramps after neck surgery were also treated with the extract. MacCallum found that the effects on the cramps varied: sometimes it worked well, in other cases nothing happened.

As the extract that MacCallum had produced did not work particularly well, he tried other methods to treat the tetany. He wrote much later that he had tested calcium's effect since "there happened to be a jar of calcium chloride in front of me on a shelf in the laboratory." This was probably not the entire truth, but rather an example of one of Louis Pasteur's aphorisms: "Chance favours the prepared mind." MacCallum's younger brother John MacCallum was a noted physiologist who had worked with Jacques Loeb for several years and published a number of reports that clarified the role of calcium in cramps. It seems unlikely MacCallum didn't know about his brother's research. The younger MacCallum had a short but productive research career (he died at the age of 30 from tuberculosis); among other things, he charted the structure and physiology of the heart muscle.

In a preliminary report from 1908 William MacCallum and his colleague Carl Voegtlin showed that the cramps that dogs suffered after having their parathyroids removed disappeared almost instantaneously when calcium was injected into the bloodstream. The effect lasted about a day and when the cramps started again they could once again be stopped by a calcium injection. They also reported that the dogs had blood calcium levels that were approximately less than half of that found in normal dogs. They felt that the effect occurred because the parathyroid had the ability to neutralise some kind of poisonous substance in the blood – the theory that Vassale had launched some ten years earlier. MacCallum therefore thought that the main function of the parathyroids was to purify the blood of harmful substances. After performing more experiments, MacCallum began to question the relevance of the toxic theory and turned instead to studying the possibility that the parathyroids might somehow play a role in the metabolism of calcium. One year earlier (in 1907), a Romanian neurologist and psychiatrist, Constantin Parhon, had published a piece in a Romanian periodical, *Revista Stiintelor Medicale*, in which he showed that cramps in dogs that had had their parathyroids removed could be stopped by administering calcium. Just as was the case with Sandström, Parhon's article in a small national journal attracted no immediate attention, nor did Parhon follow up on his experiments – another example of an important discovery not fully exploited.

By around 1910, the experiments on frogs, rats and dogs had, in principle, already solved the problems of the cramps that appeared after neck surgery; however, there were many who felt that the calcium hypothesis alone could not explain the entire phenomenon, particularly because other salts belonging to the same group as calcium (magnesium, strontium, and barium) could also stop cramps. The theory of some kind of autointoxication, where the body poisoned itself, had existed for such a long time that it was difficult for many doctors and researchers to understand that it was incorrect. Not even MacCallum was completely convinced of the direct connection between parathyroid deficiency and low calcium levels in the blood, despite the fact cramps could obviously be treated with calcium. In the beginning, he assumed that a parathyroid deficiency led to the appearance of "substances" that bound with calcium and somehow leached the calcium out of the tissues. There was no one yet who really understood the correct explanation that the parathyroids had a direct, rather than an indirect, function of maintaining the calcium levels in the blood, and MacCallum admitted that his studies had provided no absolute proof that the cause of cramps in parathyroid deficiency was solely due to low calcium levels. For the time being, one had to be satisfied with the important practical realisation that administering calcium could cure the cramps that occurred after neck surgery.

A new theory about the function of the parathyroids was proposed in 1912 by W. F. Koch. He had found that the secretion of a nitrogen-rich substance, methylguanadine, increased in the urine of dogs that had had their parathyroids removed. Koch maintained that waste materials from different proteins that had been absorbed by the body acted as toxins when the parathyroids were removed. Many people felt that the toxic substance that everyone had been looking for had finally been identified. However, MacCallum himself was not totally convinced, so he continued with new experiments on dogs. During an experiment that was just as ingenious as it was sophisticated, the circulatory systems of two dogs were joined together. One of the dogs had cramps because its parathyroids had been removed earlier, the other dog was healthy. MacCallum confirmed that the muscle cramps stopped in the dog with no parathyroids when it received blood from the healthy dog. He also showed that if the calcium was removed from the blood by dialysis, both of the dogs suffered cramps. MacCallum therefore drew the conclusion that the cramps were the result of a calcium deficiency. In spite of these experiments, many continued to pursue the theory of the significance of guanidine in the occurrence of cramps. MacCallum's frustration is apparent in the text of his *Textbook of Pathology* (1917): "Metabolism in tetany has been studied, but with unsatisfactory results, and nothing which definitely illuminates the situation has been found." At that point MacCallum gave up the idea of further trials and he published no more experiments in that area.

In an article in 1923, the Norwegian physiologist Harald Salvesen described the results of a series of experiments on dogs. Salvesen began his article by observing, "We have no certain knowledge about the function of the parathyroid." After presenting the results of his carefully executed studies, he drew the following conclusion: "These experiments show that the characteristic feature of a parathyroid deficiency is a lowering of the calcium levels in the blood, which is more pronounced when more glandular tissue has been removed. The studies show that the parathyroids control the metabolism of calcium, and in this way not only the function of the muscles and the nerves are affected, but the function of all other organs as well." This is exactly the way it worked. The decades of discussion about the role of calcium in the symptoms caused by parathyroid deficiency should have then been put aside – but it was not to be. The debate continued until the final blow to the guanidine theory was delivered in 1927 by Ralph Mayor who had developed a new method for measuring guanidine. He was able to show that no guanidine could be detected in the blood in parathyroid deficiency-induced muscle cramps.

MacCallum was finally proven right as far as the role of the parathyroids in the metabolism of calcium was concerned. His discovery had significant medical consequences and introduced a new field of research that would later provide new information about the physiology of the body. The medical historian Eran Dolev has pointed out how problematic it can be to conduct relevant laboratory experiments based on clinical observations and then attempting to transfer the results into practical medical care. In an experimental situation, researchers often have problems interpreting results, agreeing on suitable methods and concurring on what conclusions can be drawn from the experiments. A kind of ambiguous, confusing situation can arise when research hypotheses are clouded by clinical observations. Dolev regarded the experiments explaining tetany that occurred after neck surgery and the corroboration of the function of the parathyroids as illustrative examples of the difficulties of correlating animal experiments with clinical observations.

Biologists have long been aware of the fact that the biodiversity in the sea is much richer than that found in freshwater lakes and rivers. It has therefore been assumed that life on our planet first originated in the sea in the form of unicellular animals that were able to adapt to the special environment that could be found there containing sodium, calcium, and a number of other elements. These primitive animals had an internal milieu that conformed to their external environment, which is saltwater. Larger and more complex animals evolved and they required circulatory systems that could ensure a constant, nutritious environment for all of their cells. Approximately 400 million years ago certain species were able to leave their marine environment for a life on land. As a result of their developmental history, land animals have an internal milieu that corresponds to the early sea environment. The relative amounts of sodium, potassium, and calcium salts that are found in human blood exist in the same proportions as in seawater. Over time the sea has become more saline due to evaporation, and today the amounts of sodium, potassium, and calcium are three times higher in seawater than they are in our blood; however, the relative proportions between the elements are the same. Our ancestors were marine animals, and their legacy to us is the diluted saltwater circulating in our blood.

The sea, however, was not an ideal environment for specialised cellular life with a high calcium concentration of around 10 millimoles per litre. In order for primitive cells (prokaryocytes) to handle the poisonous effects of high calcium levels in the environment it was vital to develop tools to maintain very low concentrations of the calcium ion inside cells. The solution to this problem was the development of pumps that could transport the calcium ion across the cell membrane and across membranes of specialised intracellular structures (the mitochondria, the Golgi apparatus and the endoplasmatic reticulum) which could store calcium inside the cell. This created a huge (10 000-fold) calcium concentration gradient (10 millimoles per litre in the sea and 0.001 millimoles per litre inside the cell). The high concentration gradient of calcium across the cell membrane created ideal conditions for the calcium ion to be used as a signalling agent. The basic mechanism of calcium signalling is that the calcium ion is low when cells are at rest, but when an appropriate stimulus arrives there is a sudden elevation of its concentration which results in activity inside the cell. This sophisticated signalling system works like an on/off switch where the on-function introduces calcium into the fluid compartment of the cell (the cytosol) and the off-function is a mechanism that pumps calcium ions out of the cell or into calcium stores within the cell.

The calcium stores inside the cells, the ion channels that can enable calcium to enter the cells and the ion pumps that can pump calcium out of the cells are the most important mechanisms for regulating the calcium levels inside the cells. The pumps, which require energy, create a difference in voltage between the cell's intracellular and extracellular environment. This stored energy can be released much like a spark from a battery. When a specific signal reaches the cell it causes the reshaping of the cell membrane, which opens the calcium ion channels, and this allows millions of ions per second to rush through each open channel.

The cellular calcium stores can be used to regulate the concentration of calcium ions inside the cells via sophisticated signal systems and transport mechanisms. The so-called SERCA proteins help pump calcium ions into the cells' stores, the endoplasmic reticulum. Intracellular calcium levels increase when special G protein-coupled receptors (GPCRs) are activated in the cell's outer membrane, which results in the formation of inositol triphosphate (IP$_3$) which in turn activates the IP$_3$ receptors in the walls of the cell stores. This causes the cell stores to open, after which the concentration of calcium ions increases dramatically inside the cell. The elevated concentration of ions inside the cell can then trigger other tasks, such as the secretion of a hormone. When the task is finished, the ion pumps, which have the task of restoring normal calcium levels inside the cells, are activated and thereby prepare the cell for receiving signals to carry out new tasks.

In terms of developmental biology, parathyroids appeared first in amphibians (animals that can survive both on land and in water) and these glands were preserved in the animals that later migrated permanently onto land. As a remnant of the prehistoric origin of human beings, the parathyroids originate in the third and fourth branchial clefts of the human foetus, and later during foetal development they navigate down to their normal position in close proximity to the thyroid. One or more of the parathyroid glands can either get stuck on the way to their usual place, or they can travel farther than normal and end up inside of the thoracic cavity.

Fish lack parathyroids, but like humans they do have calcium-sensing receptors, (CaSR) on the cell surfaces of many different organs, such as the gills. The placement in the gills serves the purpose well as fish, like mammals, need to carefully regulate calcium levels in order to maintain the normal composition of the skeleton and surrounding layer of scales as well as for the normal function of muscles, nerve conductivity and so on.

Freshwater contains very low amounts of calcium and freshwater fish meet their calcium needs primarily from the food they eat, but also to some extent by absorbing calcium through their gills and directly through their skin. Fish in saltwater have the reverse problem as calcium levels in the sea are 3–4 times higher than the level of calcium in fish blood (fish, like most other mammals, have total calcium levels of about 2.50 millimoles per litre in the blood). Saltwater fish have a number of regulating mechanisms that ensure a constant internal calcium environment and keep the fish from being poisoned by the high calcium concentrations in seawater. They also have a unique organ located by the kidneys, consisting of the Stannius corpuscles, which lowers the concentration of calcium by secreting the hormone *hypocalcin*.

Thus saltwater fish have a well-developed regulatory system for maintaining normal calcium levels in spite of the high calcium levels in their surroundings. This is probably the developmental biological explanation as to why no parathyroid glands have ever been found in fish, even though parathyroid hormone-like peptides have been shown to exist in some fish such as trout.

Another hormone that lowers calcium concentrations and can be found in fish as well as humans is *calcitonin*. Calcitonin is produced in special cells in the human thyroid. Interestingly, there are no diseases linked to an extreme overproduction of calcitonin (e.g. in the rare form of medullary thyroid cancer) or in reduced calcitonin production (after the removal of the entire thyroid). The calcitonin in mammals is a less potent calcium reducer than that found in fish, which is why it had long been thought that human calcitonin only existed as a developmental biological remnant with no particular function or significance. Calcitonin manufactured from salmon is available as a drug that is sometimes used to lower high calcium concentrations in patients, and has been used to treat osteoporosis. Recently, however, it has been found that calcitonin probably has a role in maintaining the skeleton's structure in connection with pregnancy and lactation. During these conditions there is an increased need for calcium and calcitonin; under these circumstances calcitonin seems to contribute to the maintenance of the skeleton of pregnant women and nursing mothers. In humans, calcitonin production is increased in the female mammary glands in connection with breast-feeding, and in birds calcitonin helps in the mineralisation of eggshells.

This situation of high concentrations of calcium in the marine environments of saltwater fish is quite different from that of land mammals, where a deficient calcium intake is a constant threat. In a Western diet the main sources of calcium are dairy products such as milk and cheese. Nutritional studies have shown that many older people have a lower than recommended intake of calcium, which can contribute to the development of osteoporosis. The recommended daily allowance (RDA) for adults is 1000–1200 mg of calcium. The calcium regulating mechanisms in humans are therefore focused on maintaining calcium concentrations in the body that are higher than what is usually found in our environment.

Even though it had been understood for so long that the calcium ion was a signal substance (a "second messenger") for important cellular functions, it was not until the end of the 20th century that a method was developed to study the underlying mechanisms – what is known as calcium signalling. The actual phenomenon of fluorescence was first described in 1852 by the English physicist, Sir George Stokes, after he had found that by illuminating the mineral fluorspar or fluorite (CaF_2) with invisible ultraviolet light, the mineral could emit visible light that had a longer wavelength. A molecule fluoresces if it absorbs light of another wavelength than the light it emits. If you illuminate a fluorophore (a molecule that can fluoresce) with coloured light, it will emit light of another colour that has a different wavelength. One of the striking characteristics of the calcium ion is that when it binds with certain proteins it changes the three-dimensional structure of the complex – a circumstance that promotes the generation of fluorescence.

In the mid-1980s Roger Tsien synthesised a fluorescent substance called fura-2 that emitted light with a wavelength of 510 nanometers (nm) when it was illuminated by light with a wavelength of 380 nm. When fura-2 was saturated with calcium ions, it required light having a wavelength of 340 nm in order to have the fura-2/Ca^{2+}complex emit light with a wavelength of 510 nm. By varying the incoming light in the 340–380 nm interval he could indirectly determine the number of calcium ions in the compound. By using Tsien's extremely sensitive method, it was possible to demonstrate for the first time how calcium ions were transported and stored inside the cell. The 2008 Nobel Prize in Chemistry was awarded to Roger Tsien, Osamu Shimomura and Martin Chalfie for their "luminous discoveries" using fluorescent light.

Charting the different effects of calcium ions inside and outside of cells has revealed that these processes are more complex than anyone could have imagined when it first became possible to use molecular biology to study the body's regulation of calcium. For humans, as for other vertebrates, it is thus vital to maintain near-normal concentrations of calcium in the liquid environment surrounding the cells. The concentration of calcium ions in the blood and in other liquid spaces surrounding our cells (extracellular calcium) is rigidly maintained (about 1.1 to 1.3 millimoles per litre). In order to maintain extracellular calcium concentrations that are fairly constant, it is necessary to have mechanisms that can quickly be activated and are able to

Low ca²⁺  High ca²⁺

Before aldosterone   5 min after aldosterone

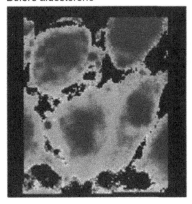
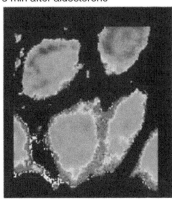

Nature reviews | Molecular cell biology

Figure 5.4 Quantification of calcium in vascular wall cells using the fluorescent protein fura-2. The left image shows a low calcium content in the cells (dark centres). Five minutes after stimulation by the hormone aldosterone, the calcium content of cells is increased (lighter colour) and even more in cell walls (stippled). (Reprinted by permission from Macmillan Publishers Ltd: Nature Reviews Molecular Cell Biology) (Online figure 1. Rapid calcium effects of aldosteronein endothelial cells. 2003, Volume 4, Issue 1.)

persist during prolonged periods of calcium deficiency. Cellular functions are extremely sensitive to abnormal concentrations of extracellular calcium. Increased nerve impulses and muscle spasms are induced by lowering the concentration of extracellular calcium by 10–20%, and lowering extracellular calcium by 50% may bring on seizures, stridorous breathing, heart failure, and death. An increase of 40–60% in extracellular calcium leads to increased thirst and drowsiness, and a 100% increase can lead to kidney failure, somnolence, coma, and death.

Nearly 50 years after Sandström's discovery, the function of the tiny parathyroid glands in maintaining the concentration of calcium in the blood had finally been established. During this process surgeons had come to realise the importance of not injuring or removing the parathyroids during neck operations. At the time most people thought that they knew everything there was to know about these glands; certainly they were vital, but if care was taken not to remove them accidentally during surgery, they were assumed to have no clinical importance. There had been reports about enlarged parathyroids and that there might be a link between the parathyroids and skeletal disease, but these facts were mainly treated as curiosities.

Yet it would soon become apparent that changes in these glands could be the cause of a serious clinical picture with medical implications that were much greater than anyone could have initially imagined. A half-century later, thousands of patients around the world were diagnosed with parathyroid disorders, and a disease had been identified that was the third most common endocrine disorder after diabetes and thyroid disorders.

Chapter 6 **Hormones and organotherapy**

The new medicine that evolved during the latter half of the 19th century attempted to make medicine more scientific by means of careful observations and systematic experimentation. This endeavour to expand medicine met with resistance from many practitioners who did not trust the newly emerging medical science and saw it as a product of elitist intellectuals lacking experience of practical work with patients. Many practitioners had poor training and relied mainly upon Hippocratic medicine that was usually limited to making a diagnosis, informing the patient of the prognosis, and prescribing general instructions for care. Most illnesses were thought to be self-regulating – either healing spontaneously or ending in death. There were many people who were convinced that most drugs were useless at best.

Advocates of the new medicine, on the other hand, tried to discover precise and effective treatments that were based on knowledge of both normal physiology and the underlying pathological changes of disease. These developments would later come to include research methodology such as randomised, controlled studies where patients were divided into separate groups by random sampling in order to study the effects of different alternative treatments.

The term "hormone" was coined by Sir Ernest Starling in a lecture at the Royal College of Physicians in London in 1905, and the discipline would later come to be known as endocrinology. The term "endocrine gland" originated in 1913 to describe an organ that secretes a chemical compound (messenger substance) into the blood that can initiate an effect in another organ or tissue. Long before the term endocrinology began to be used, endocrinological phenomena and principles had been utilised for such varied purposes as creating eunuchs for harems, being able to preserve the high tonal range of countertenors, or enhancing the flavour of the dish *Coq au Vin* by terminating

The Hunt for the Parathyroids, First Edition. Jörgen Nordenström.
© 2013 John Wiley & Sons, Ltd. Published 2013 by John Wiley & Sons, Ltd.

the sexual development of the main ingredient, young roosters or capons. As endocrinology advanced, attempts were made to understand the mechanisms governing hormonal imbalances and to find cures for hormone-related illnesses. Scientists at that time had only primitive tools, limited resources and ambiguous theories about the underlying mechanisms. In order to make advances it was necessary to integrate the knowledge of what was known within the different medical specialties including physiology, biochemistry, genetics, immunology, and molecular biology.

No other medical discipline was more contentious than the emerging field of endocrinology. While the new endocrinologists were trying to map out the foundation of the subject by patiently working with simple diagnostic tools that generally produced meagre results, there were many practitioners who were offering their patients a variety of diverse extracts made of animal tissue. In order to increase the credibility of medicine, the concept of "organotherapy" was introduced for treatments using these extracts that were claimed to be effective against almost every and any possible affliction or disease.

> "Well now, Doctor, just in confidence, I'm going to tell you something that may strike you as funny, but I believe that foxes' lungs are fine for asthma, and T.B. too. I told that to a Sioux City pulmonary specialist one time and he laughed at me – said it wasn't scientific – and I said to him, 'Hell!' I said, 'scientific' I said, 'I don't know if it's the latest fad and wrinkle in science or not', I said, 'but I get results, and that's what I am looking for's results!'"
>
> Sinclair Lewis, *Arrowsmith* (1925)

A medical discovery was made in 1891 that gave support to the cause of the organotherapy practitioners when George R. Murray demonstrated that hypothyroidism (myxedoema) could successfully be treated with thyroid extract from sheep. In the eyes of the academic doctors, this discovery was an illustration of the fact that the results of careful laboratory experiments could be converted into practical medical care, while the practitioners of organotherapy only saw this as the ultimate proof: organotherapy worked.

Parathyroid extract had been used to treat muscle cramps ever since the suspicion had arisen that the parathyroids were involved. The French physiologist Gustave Moussu was one of the first to observe that parathyroid extract from horses could remedy cramps following neck surgery on dogs. The Scottish psychiatrist C.C. Easterbrook conducted a bizarre experiment to study the effects of organotherapy. In an article in *The Lancet* from 1898, Easterbrook began by declaring that it might be of interest to compare the effects of administering parathyroid extract vs. thyroid extract as contemporary researchers had suggested that the parathyroids might have a function that was just as important as the thyroid. Easterbrook thereby became one of the first to administer parathyroid extract to humans. In an experiment that can only be described as absolutely one of the lowest watermarks in the history of medical research, Easterbrook administered parathyroid extract made from oxen to women who "suffered from insanity that either was or threatened to become chronic." These patients were not sick, rather the object of the experiment was simply to compare the effects of parathyroid extract to those of thyroid extract or, as he expressed it himself: "to spread some light on the function of the parathyroids." In these experiments the patients were forced to stay in bed during the entire observation period so that their metabolism would remain stable and thereby allow a more precise evaluation of the effects of organotherapy. The experiment began with the patients being given orally one dried ox parathyroid the first week, followed by two glands a day for two days, and then three glands a day for three days. Since this provided no discernible results, Easterbrook tried injecting the patients with ox extract, but this produced no perceivable effects either.

The advocates of the blessings of organotherapy received support for their cause when Charles Edouard Brown-Séquard, at the age of 72, reported to his astonished colleagues in a presentation at the French Academy of Sciences in 1899 that he had been "rejuvenated" after having given himself injections of an extract made from guinea pig and dog testicles. He related, "already after three days I had regained my prior vigor … my digestion and intestinal functions had improved … and I found I was able to perform mental activities more easily than I had been able to do the last few years." This news did not come from just any researcher; it came from one of France's most prominent physiologists. In 1878 Brown-Séquard had become professor of physiology after Charles Bernard at the *Collège de France*. One of his more important research contributions was made in 1856 when he proved that removal of the adrenal glands in animals was incompatible with life. The adrenal gland provided some substance that was secreted into the blood-stream that was vital for survival. Thus he introduced the method of studying the physiological effects of an organ by observing the loss of function after the removal of an organ. One could say that his studies on the adrenal gland constituted the start of endocrinology itself.

Brown-Séquard's "discovery" of the rejuvenating effects of testicle extract was good news for all who believed in organotherapy and for those who were older and wanted to regain the bodily functions that they had in their youth. Testicle transplants, serum treatments, and vaccinations with extracts became popular for a number of years among those who could afford to pay for this seemingly scientific miracle. The scientific community's reaction to the ageing physiologist's final experiment was resolutely negative. A successful research career came to a pathetic end and there were many who ridiculed him for his experiments using testicle extract.

The French-Russian doctor Serge Voronoff had been trained as surgeon in Lyon under the direction of the technically skilful and innovative Alexis Carrel. Carrel was a forerunner in transplant, vascular, and thoracic surgery, and received the Nobel Prize in 1912 for his technique of suturing blood vessels. However, he would later lose prestige because of his stance on scientific racism, and was accused of collaborating with the Vichy Régime during World War II. Voronoff worked as a surgeon in Egypt at the beginning of the 20th century, where he studied the effects of the castration of eunuchs. He felt that his studies showed that castration at an early age not only affected sexual drives, but that it also affected the muscular and psychological development of the individual and led to premature ageing. Voronoff drew the conclusion that ageing was a consequence of a diminished secretion of hormones, particularly sexual hormones. For this reason he began a program in which the testicles of chimpanzees and baboons were transplanted into the scrotums of older men in order to increase their sexual drive and to rejuvenate them mentally.

During the 1920s Voronoff's transplant operations became popular, not only for improving the sexual drive, but also for many other purported effects such as improved memory function, an increased capacity for work, and a longer life. Thousands of testicle transplants were performed around the world. Rumour has it that Pablo Picasso was one of Voronoff's patients. Voronoff established a monkey house in Menton to be able to ensure the supply of simian testicles, and a special clinic was instituted in Alger. He received applause for his operations at a meeting of the International Congress of Surgeons in London in 1923. Voronoff, who was already wealthy, saw his affluence increase. He moved into an entire floor in one of the most exclusive hotels in Paris where he was surrounded by a whole staff of personal servants, secretaries, chauffeurs, and two mistresses. His transplant business ended after the procedure was proven to be ineffective which prompted the widespread criticism of the medical community. The truth finally caught up with the fiction and Voronoff's "monkey gland business" came to be one of the century's most criticised and ridiculed cases of quackery. A reference to Voronoff's work resurfaced in 1998 in connection with the launching of Viagra, and in 1999 the journal *Nature* noted that AIDS might have been transferred from apes to humans as a result of Voronoff's transplant operations.

Mikhail Bulgakov's imaginative satire, "Heart of a Dog" (1925), is a tale that has its origin in Voronoff's transplant operations. In the story, the

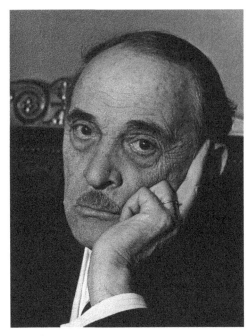

Figure 6.1 Serge Voronoff (1866–1951), Russian-French physiologist. (Reproduced with permission from Corbis)

wealthy and successful Professor Philip Philippovich in Moscow adopts a stray dog that is implanted with the testicles and the pituitary gland of a recently deceased criminal. The result is the development of a new being that has human characteristics, an animal personality and is a complete social misfit. This new hybrid starts to walk on two legs, develops fingers, begins to understand spoken language and learns to speak. He is given clothes and he adopts the name Polygraf Polygrafovich Sharik.

Three weeks after the operation, the professor's assistant, Dr. Bormenthal, writes in his laboratory notes:

> "January 12th. Put hands in pockets. We are teaching him not to swear. Whistled, 'Hey, little apple.' Sustained conversation. I cannot resist certain hypotheses: we must forget rejuvenation for the time being. The other aspect is immeasurably more important. Prof. Preobrazhensky's astounding experiment has revealed one of the secrets of the brain. The mysterious function of the pituitary as an adjunct to the human brain has now been clarified. It determines human appearance. Its hormones may now be regarded as the most

important in the whole organism – the hormones of man's image.
A new field has been opened up to science: without the aid of any
Faustian retorts a homunculus has been created. The Surgeon's
scalpel has brought to life a new human entity. Prof.
Preobrazhensky – you are a creator. But I digress . . . As stated; he can
now sustain a conversation. As I see it, the situation is as follows: the
implanted pituitary has activated the speech-centre in the canine
brain and words have poured out in a stream. I don't think that we
have before us a newly-created brain but a brain which has been
stimulated to develop. Oh, what a glorious confirmation of the theory
of evolution! Oh, the sublime chain leading from a dog to
Mendeleyev the great chemist! A further hypothesis of mine is that
during its canine stage Sharik's brain has accumulated a massive
quantity of sense-data. All the words which he used initially were the
language of the streets which he had picked up and stored in his
brain. Now as I walk along the streets I look at every dog I meet with
secret horror. God knows what is lurking in their minds."

Sharik's animal personality resulted in the life of the formerly respectable
professor becoming a veritable inferno. Finally, Professor P. saw no other
recourse than to remove the implants, after which Sharik returned to his
original canine state.

The short story was banned by the Stalinist censors since it was thought
that the dog's transformation was a metaphor for the Bolshevik Revolution.
It was not until 1988 that the story could be published in Russia.

At the 1921 meeting of the Association for the Study of Internal Secretion
(later renamed The Endocrine Society), Harvey Cushing began his
Presidential Address in the following way:

"We find ourselves embarked on the fog-bound and poorly charted
sea of endocrinology. It is easy to lose our bearings for we have, most
of us, little knowledge of seafaring and only a vague idea of our
destination. Our motives are varied. Some unquestionably follow the
lure of discovery; some are earnest colonizers; some have the spirit of
missionaries and would spread the gospel; some are attracted merely
by the prospect of gain and are running full sail before the trade
wind. Traders, adventures, even pirates are certain to follow on the
heels of exploration."

At the time Cushing was the foremost figure in American surgery after
having more or less founded the specialty of neurosurgery on his own. He
was also an authority on pituitary gland surgery and was one of the pioneers

of endocrinology. His arrogance and sharp tongue were legendary and his personality was stereotypically characteristic of a brilliant surgeon: egotistical, sarcastic, and absolutely intolerant for anything less than perfection (both in himself and in others) during operations. He was a literary personality as well and he seemed to live according to the motto, *nulla dies sine linea* (No day without a line). He was awarded a Pulitzer Prize in 1926 for a monumental biography in two thick volumes that he wrote about his former mentor and one of the icons of medicine – William Osler.

The direction of the rapidly advancing field of endocrinology was towards finding precise deviations in the hyper- and hypo-functions of the endocrine glands and administering hormones with known effects when treating specific hormonal disorders. One of the main tasks of the endocrinologists was to distance the established research world from the organotherapies that were practiced by charlatans, quacks, and poorly trained practitioners. Cushing spared no words and made a demonstrative attack on organotherapy:

> "It has been claimed that the body picks out the substance it needs and will discard the others, but this has a familiar sound of the gunshot doses of earlier days. . .Surely nothing will discredit the subject in which we have a common interest so effectively as pseudoscientific reports which find their way from the medical press into advertising leaflets, where, clearly intermixed with abstracts from researchers of actual value, the administration of pluriglandular compounds is promiscuously advocated for a multitude of symptoms, real and fictitious."

A few years later another leading endocrinologist, L. G. Rowntree, made the following statement about organotherapy: "There are still so-called pharmaceutical firms engaged in a most fraudulent exploitation of the medical profession and the public in their greed for money. They squeeze gold out of human heartaches."

Today, organotherapy has been weeded out of the medical profession but the phenomenon still lingers on. A search of "organotherapy" on the Internet returns thousands of current hits. Among other things, you can find companies that have hundreds of products made from various and sundry extracts such as brains, lungs, blood vessels, adrenal glands, hearts and skeletons (but nothing from the thyroid!), claimed to be effective for treating all kinds of different conditions such as asthma, arteriosclerosis, haemorrhoids, depression and hepatitis.

Even though the use of tissue extract is probably limited today, there are still other popular preparations that are claimed to give positive results when used to treat any number of different conditions. It has been said that the annual production of aloe vera is 420 000 litres with a turnover of $2 billion per year. However, the number of highly qualified scientific reports is quite limited. The large medical database MEDLINE contains 12 randomised, controlled studies of such treatments for different medical conditions, ten of which show no effects any better than what can be produced by using inactive substances (placebos).

Chapter 7 **The priority dispute**

During a lecture presented at the American Physiological Society in 1924, James B. Collip reported that he had succeeded in producing an active hormone from parathyroid extract. Most of the audience understood what potential significance this would have for the understanding of the physiological effects of the parathyroid glands. However some of those who were listening to Collip's lecture knew that similar results had been published earlier by another researcher named Adolph Hanson. This became the start of a long and bitter dispute over the intellectual rights to the discovery, the patent rights and the commercial exploitation of parathyroid extract. Hanson, who was a surgeon with a private practice and an amateur chemist, envisioned himself as David in a struggle against a Goliath in the form of Collip who was an established university professor with the backing of the academic research world in collaboration with the financially powerful pharmaceutical industry.

One might say that Hanson followed a long tradition of medical practitioners who had a genuine interest in research and a concern for their patients. He was the epitome of the lone doctor who was inclined to experiment which by that time had begun to be called into question by a new kind of researcher – the career researcher schooled in basic science with roots in the university institutions and the pharmaceutical industry and who was part of a research team, with specialised skills and sound academic qualifications. The last battle over the traditional way of conducting research had begun. It is true that Hanson would waltz away in victory after the strife over the patent rights to his discovery; however it would later become apparent that these new times required new solutions when it came to conducting research.

The Hunt for the Parathyroids, First Edition. Jörgen Nordenström.
© 2013 John Wiley & Sons, Ltd. Published 2013 by John Wiley & Sons, Ltd.

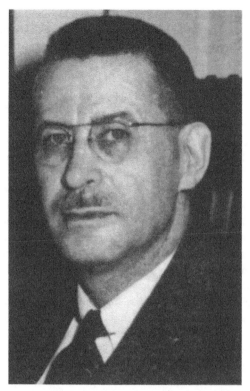

Figure 7.1 Adolph M. Hanson (1888–1959), private practice surgeon and amateur chemist, discoverer of parathyroid hormone. (Courtesy of University of Minnesota, Minneapolis, MN, USA)

Adolph Hanson had grown up in Minnesota, where he lived and worked his entire life. His family had Norwegian roots and both Adolph's father and his paternal grandfather were ministers in the Norwegian Lutheran Hauge Synod – an extremely devout church. The family identified strongly with their Norwegian fatherland, and maintained strong ties with the Norwegian farming community in Minnesota. Adolph spoke fluent Norwegian. He had been frail and sickly throughout his youth and he often needed medical care. Thus, from an early age, he began to develop an interest in medicine. Even as a young child he had performed operations on pets that he had somehow learned to anaesthetise. He successfully removed a tumour from one of the family's cats. He obviously seemed to be a born surgeon.

After having received his medical degree and finishing his training as a surgeon, he settled down and opened a practice in Faribault, Minnesota.

Hanson had only been a surgeon for three years when his father Martin Hanson, the well-known minister in the area, was stricken with a severe gallbladder inflammation. His condition worsened and it soon became apparent that an operation was necessary. Obsessively apprehensive and fearful of surgery, he insisted that he would not submit his body to any surgeon's knife except that of his son. Adolph tried desperately to get his father to agree to being operated on by one of his colleagues, but finally the young surgeon felt obliged to operate on his father. Complications arose and Adolph's father died a few weeks later. His father was 56 years old when he died and Adolph was 27. This family drama must have haunted Adolph for the rest of his life.

Hanson enlisted in the American army's medical corps when the United States entered World War I in 1917, and was stationed at a military hospital in France. During the war he gained wide experience as a neurosurgeon, and later he published a number of articles dealing with the techniques of war surgery and related issues, including how the construction of the soldiers' helmets could be improved in order to decrease the number of head injuries.

For all the destruction and chaos it wreaks, war has spurred medical advances. War theatres have since time immemorial been an important school for surgeons, something noted already by Hippocrates: "He who wishes to be a surgeon should go to war." The experience that surgeons gained during wartime indirectly came to benefit the civilian population. Dominique Jean Larrey, Napoleon's chief surgeon, created a special organisation for military medical care with medical units, mobile field hospitals ("*ambulances*") and a military medical transport system.

Historically the main threat to the lives of soldiers has not been physical injuries, but rather epidemics and infections. In 1776, George Washington had his entire army inoculated against smallpox: "Should the disease infect the Army and rage with its usual virulence, we should have more to dread from it than from the sword of the enemy." In spite of inoculation, the majority of the soldiers died from epidemics or local infections and only one out of nine soldiers that died did so from injuries on the battlefield. During World War I 'the new medicine' would be subjected to enormous challenges, particularly in the area of war surgery. The mortality rate on the Allied side was as high as 14 per 1000 soldiers during World War I, compared to 0.6 per 1000 soldiers during World War II. It was not until World War II that the number of fatalities during direct fighting was higher than the number of fatalities from other causes. Important medical developments fully utilised during World War II included penicillin, sulphur, new malaria drugs, and the use of plasma in blood transfusions for the treatment of shock.

Harvey Cushing was among those American surgeons who served in World War I. He was stationed at an American military hospital in France and was *de facto* in charge of the neurosurgery operations in the area. Medical units nearby had been instructed to send their complicated brain injuries to him. Adolph Hanson who before the war had been trained as a neurosurgeon in Philadelphia had close contacts with Cushing during the war. In actual fact, Cushing became Hanson's medical superior in neurosurgery. Cushing had a great deal of influence on Hanson and awakened his interest in research. According to Hanson, they also became good friends.

After the war, they remained in contact and Cushing offered advice on improvements to manuscripts that Hanson had sent to him. On 24th June 1919 Cushing wrote the following about Hanson's first scientific treatise:

"Dear Hanson:
I am very glad to have had your paper, but am sorry to say that it strikes me as being very casually written, nor do I feel that the title quite covers it. . . . I wonder if you realize that one has to go over and over and over again any paper before publishing it. It's a tedious business but it must be done if your communications are to be of any value. . . . Please don't think that I am finicky about this; I merely want to give you some advice and points about preparing a paper that I would give to one of my own House Officers. . . . Do go over it again as carefully as you can, and when you think you are wholly satisfied do it once more. . . . Please understand that though my criticisms may be severe they are nevertheless intended to be most friendly ones.

Sincerely yours,
H.C."

After the war Hanson returned to Faribault, which lies only about an hour's drive away from the prestigious Mayo Clinic. In spite of arduous days with his patients, Hanson wanted to do research and he enrolled at St. Olaf College where he received a Master's degree. He was given permission to do his thesis work at home so he set up a small chemistry laboratory, "The Hanson Research Laboratory," in the basement of his house. Here, he was the patron, chief chemist, assistant chemist, stenographer, bottle washer, and janitor. Most of the time not spent caring for his patients, Hanson spent in his laboratory. His children have later related that they helped out by preparing different organs in the kitchen meat grinder, and that they were often served leftovers from their father's animal experiments for dinner. Their mother Lucille's culinary skills came in handy here, for she would heighten the flavour – either by frying the organ extracts in butter (which was the tastier option) or by serving it with cream gravy.

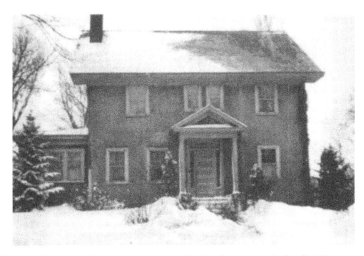

Figure 7.2 Hanson Research Laboratory at the family home in Faribault, Minnesota. (Courtesy of University of Minnesota, Minneapolis, MN, USA)

Hanson had experience with goitre surgery from both his surgical training and his own patients. He was well aware that the removal of, or injury to, the parathyroids during neck surgery could lead to cramps. In the autumn of 1922 he began chemically analyzing the parathyroids of beef cattle. He spent long hours at a local slaughterhouse, and at best could get hold of 8–12 glands at the same time for use in his experiments. He analyzed the different organic and inorganic substances in the extract. He performed unconventional experiments out of his sheer desire for experimentation, and discovered that boiling the parathyroids in hydrochloric acid produced an abundant precipitate that he called 'Hypochloric X.' He assumed that the extract contained some kind of active substance. Later Hanson described how he felt when he was ridiculed for his method of boiling the tissue in hydrochloric acid which ought to have destroyed all hormones according to what was believed at the time. In his own defense, he claimed, "In order to tackle unknown problems, a man needs a little less chemical knowledge and more humility … because I knew so little chemistry I boiled the glands in a strong mineral acid for two hours to isolate the hormone. What real chemist would ever have done that?"

Hanson himself had no resources for testing the physiological effects of his extract, but got in touch with another researcher, A. B. Bell at the University of North Dakota, who was willing to conduct the animal experiments. In spite of protests from the local ethics committee (!), they obtained four dogs that had their parathyroids removed. The resulting cramps that the dogs suffered could be treated to some extent by administering 'Hypochloric X', and Bell reported with great enthusiasm that the extract contained an active substance.

Considering the subject, Hanson published his results in an obscure publication: *The Military Surgeon*. By doing this, he repeated the same mistake that Ivar Sandström had made earlier, not to make his results immediately available to the researchers who had a particular interest in the subject.

It was evident that further experiments with 'Hypochloric X' were necessary. One of America's most prominent chemists, Edward Kendall, worked at the nearby Mayo Clinic. In 1914 at only 28 years of age, he had isolated thyroxine – the main hormone produced in the thyroid. Kendall later isolated cortisone ('Substance X'), and he shared the 1950 Nobel Prize for this discovery with Philip Hench and Tadeus Reichstein. Kendall performed several experiments with Hanson's extract: "We have tried the material on one or two cases here, but have seen no physiological effect." Other researchers that Hanson had contacted performed experiments with dogs that were described as "promising, but not conclusive." Hanson treated some of his patients with the extract and reported that it was effective for treating chronic inflammatory conditions such as stomach and leg ulcers, urinary infections, and bone infections.

James Collip represented a new, different kind of researcher than Hanson. He was a career scientist with a solid biochemical background and held an academic position allowing him to perform full-time basic scientific research. He also had access to an academic network and substantial financial resources. Collip had previously earned a solid reputation as a researcher after having taken part in the isolation of insulin. When Frederick Banting and John Macleod received the 1923 Nobel Prize for the discovery of insulin, it was the spark that ignited one of the most famous disputes over the intellectual rights to a discovery. Banting was furious about the decision that Macleod got a share in the prize. Banting felt that Macleod had not actively contributed to the discovery and that his role had primarily been to provide resources for carrying out the experiments.

Those who defended Macleod conceded that Banting had come up with the idea of extracting the active substance from the pancreatic gland after having first removed the enzyme trypsin (which would have neutralised the insulin), but that he was a surgeon who lacked scientific training and resources to carry out the experiments. They contested that the basic idea he had was of no relevance to the commercial production of insulin. Without Macleod's support, Banting's idea probably would have remained a hypothetical possibility. At first Banting refused to accept the award, but changed his mind because of pressure from the Canadian government who felt that it

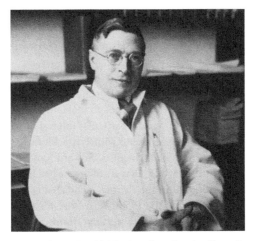

Figure 7.3 James B. Collip (1892–1965), Canadian chemist. Photo from around 1930 when Collip was a professor of biochemistry at McGill University, Montreal. (Source: Library and Archives Canada/Lawrence Johnston Burpee fonds/C-037756.)

would look bad if the first North American to be awarded the Nobel Prize refused to accept this acknowledgement. Banting maintained that his close colleague Charles Best was the rightful person to share in the prize and, for that reason, he gave half of his prize money to Best. Macleod made the same gesture and shared his award with Collip. The dispute between the members of the research team was conducted in public and it never really came to an end. Paranoid manoeuvers, suspicions, rivalry and rumour mongering were just some of the ingredients of this conflict in which the larger scientific community generally was reluctant to get involved. One researcher made the comment that, "In insulin there is glory enough for all."

Collip had played a key role in the isolation of insulin by developing a method to increase the purity of the pancreatic extracts from animals, and by developing a method to measure the effect of insulin based on its effect on lowering blood sugar levels in rabbits. He was one of the co-authors of the primary publication on the discovery of insulin and was a co-owner of the patent granted for the method of its isolating. The Nobel Committee did not investigate Collip's role more closely because he had not been nominated and therefore, according to the statutes, he could not be considered for the prize. Several researchers who later studied the story that led up to the discovery of insulin have concluded that Collip's contributions could have merited a share of the prize, and that the trio Banting, Best and Collip were perhaps the constellation most worthy of the prize. Collip lay low during the entire debate: "The part which I was able to contribute subsequently to the work of the team was only that which any well-trained biochemist could be expected to contribute."

In mid-1924, Collip began his studies of parathyroid tissue. And then things really began to happen. After his work with insulin, Collip had a great deal of experience in isolating substances from extracts and, in addition, he had the necessary resources from the royalties of insulin sales. He used large amounts of tissue, usually 75–100 parathyroid glands from oxen for the preparation of his extract. His first publication was based on tests using as many as 35 dogs that had undergone parathyroidectomies. Collip's unconventional methods, like Hanson's, were based upon extraction by using a warm hydrochloric acid solution. His extract was purer and more active than Hanson's, and the physiological effects were more apparent: the extract could prevent tetany due to parathyroid deficiency in dogs for several months and the cramps returned if the extract was no longer administered. Collip also successfully treated a young boy with tetany by using the new hormone, and with his experiments he was able to demonstrate that giving large doses of the hormone caused von Recklinghausen's disease of bone. Collip named the new hormone parathyroid hormone (PTH).

At first, the active principle of the extract was determined by evaluating the biological effects through observing the extract's ability to prevent tetany in laboratory animals after the parathyroids had been removed. Of course, it was complicated to determine the biological activity this way, so Collip and his colleague Clark devised a method to determine the concentration of calcium in the blood. This method became the standard technique for determining blood calcium concentrations in most laboratories over the next 40 years. This was a major step forward – even though it was an indirect method since there was still no method available for measuring the actual concentration of the hormone itself – and it was now possible to determine reliably the effects of the extract. By measuring calcium levels, Collip could then study both the effects of parathyroid deficiency and excess. He discovered that the calcium concentrations in the blood could become abnormally high when large doses of extract were administered, and that dogs could become apathetic, unconscious and sometimes even die as a result of overdoses. Collip warned repeatedly that overdosing the extract could be lethal. He was also careful to point out the importance of not extrapolating the use of the extract to areas other than to treat parathyroid deficiency after surgery.

Even before Collip had begun to publish his findings, he had contacted Eli Lilly, the pharmaceutical company he collaborated with on insulin. By the time Collip published his findings in prestigious American, British and Canadian periodicals, Eli Lilly produced a commercial extract, Para-Thor-Mone.

All of these events happened in rapid succession – less than two years had passed between Collip's first tests and the delivery of a commercial product to market. Surgeons around the world now had access to a drug that could be used to treat parathyroid deficiency after neck surgery. However, it turned out that the extract was not particularly effective for the treatment of parathyroid hormone deficiency in the long term as the effect of the treatment gradually lessened – a kind of immunity or resistance to the extract developed over time.

Initially Hanson was happy about Collip's reports that supported his original hypothesis, but his feelings soon changed to disappointment and anger over the fact that Collip had not given him the acknowledgment he felt was his due. Hanson wrote a number of letters to Cushing where he related the research developments and his frustration over the lack of recognition from Collip. In a letter dated 11th April 1925, Cushing wrote:

> "My dear Hanson:
> I am distressed to know that you are disturbed by the fact that
> someone may have stolen your thunder. The world, as you know, is
> unjust and questions of priority are difficult to settle. As a matter of
> fact, I don't believe anyone has ever been granted priority in any
> struggle who has made a personal struggle for it. Most of us do our
> scientific work with a far different object in view than eliciting
> applause. If we happen to make a good strike and it happens to be
> applauded, so much better, but no one has ever been applauded or
> been given credit if he set out to demand it.
>
> What I think I would do if I were you and if you think that
> Dr. Collip has overlooked your work, would be to write him a friendly
> note and send him your papers, and ask him whether he was aware of
> it, but I would not let him know that your feelings are hurt.
>
> A great many men, for example, were on the edge of the discovery
> of insulin and might well enough have put in a claim for priority over
> Banting, but Banting after all was the man who made it all clear to
> everybody, and I don't believe that anyone, even though he may have
> spent his lifetime on diabetes, really begrudges him his discovery. You
> show fine spirit in tackling this difficult problem and your real
> friends will appreciate this whether or not the work receives the
> plaudits it deserves.
>
> Always sincerely yours,
> H.C."

These lines from one of that era's most successful and prestigious surgeons at Harvard Medical School could not have been much consolation to a

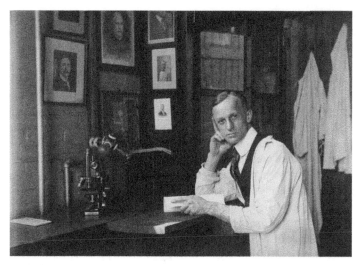

Figure 7.4 Harvey Cushing (1869–1939), American neurosurgeon and endocrinologist. (Used with permission from The Alan Mason Chesney Medical Archives of the The Johns Hopkins Medical Institutions)

little-known surgeon and private practitioner, performing research alone in a small town in the Minnesota countryside. On 15th April 1925, Hanson wrote Cushing a letter in reply:

> "This is the one big thing in my life and it means everything to me to be given credit for my discovery. You will realize, I am sure, that I consider it no trifling matter when I am wrapped up in heart and soul. . . . It is far more than a question of money. It is immortality."

Cushing's reference to Banting was well-founded since there were many similarities to Hanson's situation and Banting's early career: both were surgeons and both lacked scientific training and a knowledge of biochemistry. The main difference, and one that was crucial for the final result, was that Banting had successfully established collaborative relationships with leading academic researchers and had gained access to the laboratory resources that were necessary for the completion of the project. In principle, Hanson had similar potential opportunities practically in his own backyard at the Mayo Clinic. Hanson was good friends with the influential Mayo brothers who had been guests at the Hanson home on several occasions. In addition one of the most prominent biochemists and endocrinologists of the times, Edward Kendall, was at the Mayo Clinic. Despite these similarities, Banting received the Nobel Prize and was knighted, while Hanson returned to his medical practice and remained forgotten for the most part, in spite of the fact that he had developed an idea and conducted a research project that might have been very successful if it had been organised differently. Sometimes the difference between success and failure is quite small.

We do not know whether Hanson wrote a letter to Collip as Cushing had urged him to do; however, Collip denied ever knowing anything about Hanson's early experiments, and he never referred to Hanson's work other than in a rare footnote. Hanson felt that Collip had plagiarised his research work and was disappointed that the academic establishment, "Organised Medicine," had not credited him with being the originator of the process for isolating the active parathyroid extract. He also thought that he had been deceived by Eli Lilly since he had contacted them early on about the commercial production of his extract.

Hanson's involvement with organotherapy probably played a significant role in his lack of recognition. At the time, serious researchers tried to distance themselves from organotherapy in every possible way. As newly elected president of *The Association for the Study of Internal Organs*, Collip's declaration that monkey glands were a lot of humbug – in reference to Voronoff's transplant operations – made big news headlines. In certain respects, perhaps Hanson was a pawn in the veritable crusade against organotherapy that some of the leading endocrinologists ran in order to maintain the credibility of scientifically based hormone therapy. What did not speak in Hanson's favour was the fact that he maintained that his extract had a wider field of application than just being a replacement for parathyroid deficiency after neck surgery. In 1924 Hanson wrote in an article in *The Military Surgeon* stating that he did not claim that the cure was "a cure-all.... no matter how remarkable the action may be in some cases." In a letter to a colleague Hanson wrote: "the struggles, the repeated defeats, the forlorn hope in a basement laboratory, rudely equipped, brings out the very bowels of the earth, what millions of dollars and superior minds have failed to do.... It will benefit hundreds of thousands. It is a real SERVICE to humanity."

Hanson also isolated a thymus extract (sweetbread extract) that he named *Karkinolsin*. He used the preparation for the treatment of cancer and he published case studies of some patients in whom he observed reductions in tumour sizes. However, Cushing cautioned him about this project in a letter dated 25th February 1924:

> "Let me warn you against getting your name attached to any therapeutic measure for carcinoma. Hundreds of men better than you and I have lost their reputations utterly by putting out something of

this kind while it was half-baked and when they thought that they had some very surprising results. A great number of things may modify the progress of malignant disease. Indeed, malignant disease has been known to disappear spontaneously. But I do not wish to discourage you, merely to give you a fatherly word of advice.

Always sincerely yours,

H.C."

Hanson began collaboration with the Parke-Davis pharmaceutical company. In March 1925 he submitted a patent application and at the same time transferred the rights of use for his parathyroid extract to the company.

A statement from the U. S. Patent Bureau in November 1927 verified that three other applications had been received besides Hanson's, namely Collip's, Lewis Berman's from Columbia University in New York and Joseph Morell's from the Swan-Meyer Company. Hanson and Berman were the two who had the earliest claims of priority which meant that Collip's and Morell's applications were denied review. While Hanson had the earliest documentation that the active properties of the extract could prevent the occurrence of cramps in cases of parathyroid deficiency, Berman thought that he should be given priority for the discovery since he had been the first to demonstrate the ability of the extract to increase calcium levels. Berman felt Hanson had not documented an awareness of the extract's physiological effects. The Patent Bureau established that it was unnecessary for the claim to discovery that the inventor should understand the reason why the discovery served its purpose, or whether or not the inventor had any knowledge of the chemical, physical or physiological characteristics that the extract possessed. The main thing was that the extract worked, and Hanson had been the first to prove that.

This ruling meant that Hanson was granted priority for the invention, but the next question was whether he could obtain the patent rights. According to the U. S. patent laws, a patent application has to be registered within two years of the date when the discovery was made known to the public. Hanson's original paper had been published in March 1925, his patent application was dated 30th March 1927, and the Patent Bureau deemed that the patent could not be granted. Hanson requested a reconsideration of the decision and, paradoxically enough, he was forced to maintain that the only purpose of his original publication, the basis for his priority claim, had been to prove that there were protein components in the extract, and that at that point he had not known that the same method could be used to produce parathyroid hormone. His request was denied at first, but was later accepted. After years of litigation, Hanson was granted both the formal priority for the discovery and the patent rights to the isolation process. Hanson commented on this recognition in the following way:

> "It seems that I am about to receive the credit for being the first to reach the North and the South poles of the Parathyroid problem as Amundsen did with the earth and his dogs. Others reached them too, but he was the first one there. He was a crude explorer, but he got there, and he got there first."

For Hanson, who had much of his identity linked to his Norwegian heritage, it must have felt good to be able to refer to the explorer Roald Amundsen's achievements. Amundsen had undertaken several spectacular expeditions: he discovered the so-called Northwest Passage from the Atlantic Ocean to the Pacific Ocean via the Canadian interior, and he was the first to reach the South Pole.

In 1933 Hanson received a gold medal from the Minnesota State Medical Association, which was noted in the local newspapers:

> "Dr. Adolph Hanson [was presented] a gold medal in recognition of his achievement which stands out in the minds of scientists in a peculiarly romantic fashion because it was achieved alone in a little basement laboratory in Faribault."

William Mayo presented the medal and made special note of the fact that Hanson had signed over all future royalty rights to the Smithsonian Institution:

> "The line between the man of business and the man of science is clear cut. Dr. Hanson waged a long fight in the courts to obtain legal title to his parathyroid findings. Consider now the admirable use to which the doctor has devoted the results of this courtroom victory. Instead of profiting by his legal patent royalties, Dr. Hanson has in fact donated them in perpetuity to the furtherance of research."

Eventually Collip became a master of the isolation of hormones from tissue extract, and after finishing his research on the parathyroids he went on to isolate hormones from the prostate, the placenta, the ovaries, and the pituitary gland. Many significant discoveries resulted from his research work and he was nominated for a Nobel Prize on six occasions during the years 1928–1951. In the evaluation reports, it was stressed that Collip's work was of major importance, and in certain respects it had been a defining moment in the development of parathyroid hormone. However, it was also pointed out that when it came to the question of the operating mechanisms of different hormones, Collip often stopped halfway and also that Hanson was the first to isolate the active substance in the parathyroids. The overall assessment was that Collip's work was not exemplary enough for the prize.

Collip probably missed the chance of receiving the Nobel Prize because he had not been nominated for the discovery of insulin. His research strategy was to concentrate on unsolved problems and, as he often said himself, "to skim the cream off the milk" and then quickly move on to the next problem – a strategy that can hardly be expected to lead to a Nobel Prize. He simply tried to cover too large an area in too short a time, and he was more interested in the practical applications of biochemistry than theoretical scientific development.

The endocrinologist Paul Munson wrote the following about the dispute between Collip and Hanson:

> "[Even though Hanson was awarded priority in the discovery]
> Collip's work was more readily accepted by the scientific community
> because, to some extent, the growing profession of endocrinology
> preferred to accept the contributions of a biochemistry professor,
> with a grand discovery already to his credit, over that of a small-town
> practitioner and amateur chemist."

Producing an extract was not enough for the medical establishment. The discoverer also had to understand what the extract contained and provide evidence of the physiological effects. Being able to receive scientific recognition requires more than just reaching the North and South Poles. One had also to realise that one had been there and be able to prove it.

The focus of academic research shifted from the hospital bed to the laboratory when the criteria for proving the effects of a hormone shifted from clinical to physiological and chemical effects. Endocrinologists began collaborating with the pharmaceutical industry in order to obtain resources to produce new hormones and have their effects tested clinically. The royalties from successful products could be used by the researchers for new research projects. In principle, it had become impossible for the lone researcher to develop new drugs. The research of the new era demanded researchers who were scientifically well-educated and usually employed by universities, and maintained good contacts with the industry. Medical research had evolved into a new phase. The era of the solitary enthusiasts with no solid scientific background and minimal resources for research had come to a close.

In the beginning, there were great hopes that the parathyroid hormone would have many medical applications. Three different pharmaceutical companies (Lilly, Parke-Davis and Squibb) sold extracts for some time. The intended areas of application, namely the treatment of non-specific tetany conditions and of parathyroid hormone deficiency following neck surgery, turned out to be very limited. Over time, the effect on the patients treated with repeated injections of the hormone lessened.

The hopes that the hormone could be used in other non-specific applications, such as a pick-me-up to increase energy or as a restorative tonic, were also abandoned. This led to the extract having only a single significant use as a tool for studying the physiology of the parathyroids. As will be shown later, at the beginning of the 21st century the interest in parathyroid hormone as a drug would reappear.

Chapter 8 **Immortal patients**

In the history of medicine there are a few patients who have become world-renowned because they received treatments linked to epoch-making medical advances. These patients include Gilbert Abbott (first use of anaesthesia, 1846); Leonard Thompson (the first diabetic treated with insulin, 1922); Albert Alexander, a policeman from Oxford (first treatment with penicillin, 1941); Mrs. Gardner (the first cortisone treatment, 1948); Richard Herrick (first successful kidney transplant, 1954); Lewis Washkansky (first heart transplant, 1967); and Louise Joy Brown (the first test-tube baby, 1978). There are also two such patients in the history of the parathyroids: sea captain Charles Martell from New York and tram driver Albert Jahne from Vienna.

The road to understanding the diseases of the parathyroid glands and their importance can be said to have diverged in two directions. One was the German, traditional, anatomical-pathological school of medicine (what happened, what was the problem?). The other, more modern school, represented by the American physiological-biochemical school that endeavoured to understand mechanisms and connections (how things work and why?). Both schools would contribute to charting the function and significance of the parathyroids, each through their own methods.

The Irish Sea, 9th April 1917. The Atlantic Ocean was in uproar, lightning illuminated the sky and waves as high as houses poured over the *SS New York*. Since its departure from New York on the 31st of March, the passenger ship had been having a difficult time crossing to Europe, but now was caught in a severe storm. The ship broke through the high waves and rolled violently back and forth on the rough seas. The long journey from America to Europe was almost over and the crew and the passengers caught sight of land far-off in the distance as they crested the waves. Three days earlier the United States had declared war on the German Empire and World War I was entering a

The Hunt for the Parathyroids, First Edition. Jörgen Nordenström.
© 2013 John Wiley & Sons, Ltd. Published 2013 by John Wiley & Sons, Ltd.

decisive phase. Europe was in a military and humanitarian morass. Transatlantic crossings at that time were life and death adventure. German submarines, fighter planes and mines were threats to both Allied and neutral ships. England, which had relied on its naval supremacy on the high seas from the time of Nelson had come to realise that emerging submarine technology would play a pivotal role. The new German submarines proved to be deadly weapons.

There were two famous people onboard the *SS New York*. One was a decorated military officer in the U.S. Navy; the other was a newly graduated naval cadet. Admiral William Sims was on his way to England together with an aide to discuss a unified command for the Allied navies. Earlier Sims had untiringly criticised the poorly armed American navy, which resulted in the U. S. Navy building the most powerful battleships in the world at that time. After the United States entered the war, Sims was placed in command of America's naval forces in Europe. He later received several of the highest honours that an American could achieve: a naval destroyer named after him, the Pulitzer Prize for his book on the naval history of World War I, *Victory at Sea* (1921), and his portrait on the cover of *Time Magazine*.

The other person, who later became a medical celebrity, was Charles Martell. He was a 22-year old cadet in the merchant marines who had graduated the previous year from the Massachusetts Nautical Training School at the head of his class. In photographs from the time he appeared as a stately young man with a steady gaze smiling into the camera. He had hopes of a bright future but he could not have conceived that he would ever become famous, and certainly not the reason for it.

Just as the passengers on the *SS New York* caught sight of Liverpool in the distance, an enormous explosion was heard causing the 10 000 ton ship to crack wide open. Most of the passengers were in the dining room finishing their dinner. Many fell down, chairs overturned, glasses and bottles toppled over or were shattered. The emergency alarm sounded throughout the entire ship and everyone rushed up towards the deck to the lifeboats that they had previously been assigned. Mayday signals were sent over the radio and were immediately picked up in the Liverpool harbour and by the ships in the vicinity. The worst was feared: a German submarine had caught sight of the ship and had fired a torpedo. Everyone on board knew that if that was the case, there was a great risk that a second torpedo would soon be fired to finish off the ship. But no new explosion followed, it appeared that the ship had hit a mine that was floating adrift. The explosion had ripped open a gaping hole on the port side of the ship and Captain J. T. Roberts ordered everyone into the lifeboats. The sinking of the Titanic, almost to the day five years earlier, had resulted in more stringent safety regulations and had made

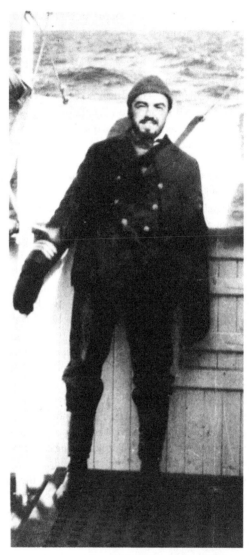

Figure 8.1 Charles Martell, one of the first patients diagnosed with hyperparathyroidism. He underwent seven operations before a pathologically enlarged parathyroid gland was removed. (Reproduced with permission, Massachusetts General Hospital, Boston, MA, USA)

training evacuation manoeuvers obligatory for transatlantic crossings. Yet rescuing the 60 passengers was not easy. It was extremely difficult to lower the lifeboats in the raging storm and one was almost broken to pieces by the violently rotating propeller on the starboard side that had ended up spinning in the air above the water's surface. The weather worsened and a snowstorm ensued. In the harsh winds the small lifeboats bobbed up and down like corks on the violent sea. The passengers were picked up by ships that had rushed to their rescue, and all were saved in the end. The SS *New York* was able to limp the remaining 35 nautical miles and docked in Liverpool. Charles Martell was certainly happy to have the solid ground of Liverpool beneath his feet. Sims and his aide were met on the dock by Admiral Hope from the British Admiralty and they were taken by a specially chartered train to London.

Charles Martell survived the mine accident and would also survive World War I serving as a navigation officer on American troop transport ships. After the war ended, Martell would encounter a new and different kind of battle. This time it was not a matter of fighting identifiable soldiers from an enemy country on a battlefield or on the open sea; it was guerilla warfare against an internal, invisible adversary whose character would only be revealed later on. Martell's personal war would last 14 years, and he would fight a courageous battle, he would have his metabolism studied by some of the most prominent researchers and clinical endocrinologists of the times, he would undergo a total of seven operations and have his disease described in the most prestigious medical journals, including three separate articles with a total of 30 pages in the influential *Journal of Clinical Investigation*. He would come to lose his own internal war, yet he would help us understand a disease that would be shown to be more common than anyone could have imagined.

By the mid-1920s, the function of the parathyroids in regulating the calcium concentration in the blood had been established, and it had been shown that the muscle cramps that were caused by a parathyroid deficiency after goitre surgery could be treated by administering calcium. Yet there were also other reports about changes in the parathyroids as a result of skeletal disease. This was the situation when "Albert J." arrived on the scene: divergent observations, unclear connections, and heated debates.

The second patient who would become famous was Viennese tram driver, Albert Jahne, also known as "Albert J." He was 38 years old in 1925 when he was admitted to the Second Surgical Clinic – Billroth's old clinic – at the *Allgemeine Krankenhaus*. Over the previous five years he had been suffering from fatigue and skeletal pain which had led to his retirement on disability. An X-ray examination showed a weakened, cystic and deformed skeleton. The diagnosis was certain: Albert J. had von Recklinghausen's bone disease (*osteitis fibrosa cystica*). When he was admitted to the hospital he had so much skeletal pain that he could not walk, sit or stand. He was emaciated; he had kidney stones and such a high secretion of calcium residue in his urine that sediment would build up in his bedpan. Attempts had been made to treat him with mercury (for syphilis, which he had contracted in his youth), cod liver oil, "electric treatments," and mud baths. Thyroidin and Parathyroidin (thyroid and parathyroid extracts) had been tested as well. The use of all these therapeutic modalities showed that the doctors were fumbling in the dark with no clear understanding of either the cause of the illness or what mechanisms were involved in the patient's ever more desperate condition. It was absolutely certain that he was going to die from his disease unless something was done. But what to do? It had been suspected for about 20 years that there could be some kind of functional disorder in the parathyroids, but how did the high blood calcium concentrations, the skeletal changes and the parathyroid dysfunction fit together? No one had a clue, and no one knew what treatment would have been appropriate.

In the case of Albert J.'s disease, there was a strong suspicion that he might have a parathyroid disorder, but was it hypofunction or hyperfunction? In order to investigate whether there was a deficiency, four parathyroid glands were transplanted onto the patient's abdominal wall. The glands had been removed from a patient who had died in an accident and been taken to the emergency ward. The parathyroid transplant did not improve Albert J.'s condition. The question arose as to whether the transplant was functioning (it was known that this was not always the case); or was the reason for the patient's condition actually an increased activity of the parathyroids?

Felix Mandl was one of the surgeons at the clinic and was used to taking the bull by the horns. A parathyroid operation seemed to be Albert J.'s only chance. Mandl assumed that if the cause was not hypofunction of the parathyroids; the reason could perhaps be a hyperfunction? On 20th July 1925, Mandl performed an operation on Albert J. using a local anaesthetic and he soon found and removed a yellowish brown, almond-shaped parathyroid tumour on the left side of the neck. The tumour measured $25 \times 15 \times 12$ mm, which was definitely larger than a normal gland and the microscopic examination showed diseased tissue. Mandl reported later: "We excitedly followed the course of events and could soon establish that the patient's condition improved markedly very soon after the operation." This description was no exaggeration. The patient's urine was completely clear after 5 days and the calcium levels in his urine sank to less than 1/5 of what they had been before the operation. He gained weight and after a while he could stand and walk using a cane. An X-ray examination a few months after the operation showed that the density of his skeleton had increased considerably. A change of almost biblical proportions had been achieved: an invalid patient had been brought in on a stretcher and he was able to walk out of the hospital on his own two feet. A dying patient had been cured.

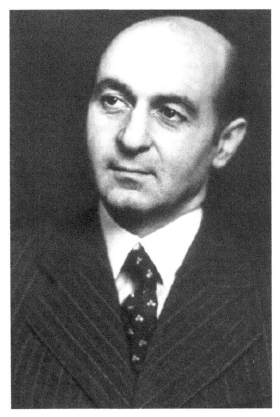

Figure 8.2 Felix Mandl (1892–1957) conducted in 1925 the first operation
for hyperparathyroidism at the *Allgemeine Krankenhaus* in Vienna. (Picture Archive,
Austrian National Library)

As a result of the operation, important insights were gained into the cause of this
disease and its clinical consequences: the skeletal changes in von Recklinghausen's
disease were due to a parathyroid tumour and not vice versa as the advocates of
the compensation theory had believed. Mandl reported on Albert's case just
a few months after the operation and its successful results became widely
recognised among medical practitioners in Europe, resulting in many surgeons
operating on parathyroids. In 1927 one of Mandl's colleagues in Vienna, E. Gold,
operated on another patient with von Recklinghausen's bone disease who was
also found to have an enlarged parathyroid gland, and he coined the name
hyperparathyroidism (i.e. an over-productive parathyroid gland) – the name
still used to denote the condition of increased parathyroid activity, elevated calcium concentrations in the blood, and one or more enlarged parathyroid glands.

After several years of continuing improvement, Albert J.'s condition began to worsen and the calcium levels in his blood became elevated again. He had a relapse of the disease. In October 1933, Mandl performed a new operation, but this time he could find no pathological parathyroids, thus it was an unsuccessful operation. Albert's condition continued to decline and three years after the second operation he died of kidney failure. The final course of events of his disease had not been prevented, but the first operation had given Albert almost 10 relatively symptom-free years, and important knowledge had been acquired that would come to benefit other patients.

At about the same time that Albert J. was being operated on in Vienna, Charles Martell fell ill on the other side of the Atlantic with a clinical picture typical of *osteitis fibrosa cystica*. His skeleton had been leached of much of its calcium, he had suffered multiple fractures and he had kidney stones. The course of Martell's illness would be even more complicated than Albert J.'s and the doctors and researchers who tried to treat him and understand his disease would come to admire Martell for his courage. He began to actively take part in the different experiments that were performed, and in actual fact he became both patient and researcher. Martell had been studied by some of the most prominent researchers in the United States early in his illness. One of them, Eugene DuBois in New York, observed that Martell had elevated calcium levels in his blood and a weakened skeleton. Since Collip's studies had shown that the administration of large amounts of parathyroid extract had caused elevated levels of calcium in the blood, it was suspected that Martell's illness was due to an overproduction of parathyroid hormone. Without having any knowledge of the successful operation on Albert J. in Vienna almost one year earlier, it was decided to perform a parathyroid operation on Martell. Yet in May 1926, no enlarged parathyroid glands were found when the operation was performed, and a new operation was undertaken a few months later because the patient's condition continued to worsen. No diseased enlarged gland was found the second time either. Naturally enough, the conclusion was drawn that perhaps Martell's skeletal disease was not caused by parathyroid disease at all.

The suspicion that Charles Martell was suffering primarily from an enlarged parathyroid gland became stronger as time went on, since more reports had appeared of cases with a clinical picture that was similar to Martell's, where it had been possible to remove an enlarged parathyroid gland by operating, often with remarkable results. Martell's condition became more worrisome and further studies of his metabolism were needed in order to determine whether the underlying cause really was an enlarged parathyroid gland. Martell was referred to Joseph Aub in Boston for a detailed analysis of his calcium metabolism.

Aub had developed a programme to treat lead poisoning based on the premise that lead and calcium were handled by the body in similar ways. Lead was stored in the same place in the body as calcium, and by increasing the urinary calcium excretion one could also increase the secretion of lead. In the 1920s lead poisoning had become a major problem among workers in many industries due to its wide use in electric cables, water pipes, batteries, paints, ammunition, bottle caps and cans, etc. Lead has no functional role in the body and is toxic because it has characteristics that are similar to those of several other biologically important metals such as calcium, iron and zinc. Lead poisoning can cause injury to a number of different organ systems and cause nerve damage, stomach pains (painter's colic), drowsiness or abnormal elation, kidney damage, anaemia, and infertility. The treatment developed by Aub involved giving large amounts of calcium to patients with acute lead poisoning, causing an increase in the secretion of lead in the urine as well as an increase in the storage of lead in the skeleton. After the acute symptoms had disappeared, and in cases of chronic lead poisoning, the patients were put on a calcium-free diet. After Collip's parathyroid extract became available, it was used to remove the lead that had been stored in the skeleton. Thus Para-Thor-Mone could be used not only for the treatment of parathyroid deficiency but also to treat chronic lead poisoning.

The use of lead in the auto industry was widespread: it was used for speeding up the vulcanisation of rubber for tyres, in spray painting, in battery production and in welding. Many of the new cases of lead poisoning that appeared at the time were due to the expanding automobile market and increased competition between the different auto makers. For many years Ford had held a dominant position with their relatively simple Model T with its weak motor. General Motors (GM) tried to take greater market share by launching their flagship Cadillac, with new models that were more comfortable, more exclusive and faster than the Model T. In order to increase the motor's performance, GM increased the cylinder compression in their engines. This created a problem since the gasoline-air mixture tended to ignite too soon and caused knocking in the motor. The knocking decreased the performance and could damage the motor. The solution to the problem was to add lead to the gasoline in the form of tetraethyl-lead. Engine performance improved significantly by using leaded gasoline and in 1922 several of the cars in the Indianapolis 500 had leaded gas in their tanks. This was a marketing success: the cars using leaded gasoline won the first, second and third prizes. A huge market for leaded gas arose and GM, Standard Oil and DuPont started a joint company, the Ethyl Corporation, to produce the new super gasoline.

The problem with tetraethyl-lead is that it is a volatile substance that is highly toxic because it can easily be absorbed in the body through the lungs and the skin. Hundreds of workers at the Ethyl Corporation's production plant in New Jersey suffered lead poisoning shortly after the production of the new gasoline mixture began. Ten employees died and others became psychotic and spent the rest of their lives confined to mental institutions. The workers called the plant "The House of Butterflies", which referred to the psychotic employees who tried to brush away the insects that they hallucinated covered their clothes. It was an environmental scandal; yet, the company maintained that there was no proof linking lead to the illnesses the workers were suffering. The company agreed to finance research about the problem on two conditions. Firstly, that the authorities refrained from publicly commenting on the matter until the experiments were completed and second, that authorities pledged not to use the word "lead," but to only use the trademark "ethyl" to describe the product. The funding of the research was granted on the condition that all manuscripts be sent to the company for review, comments and approval prior to publication. Over a period of eight months different laboratory animals were exposed 188 times to tetraethyl-lead, half of them for three hours and the other half for six hours each time. No hazardous effects were found in the laboratory animals and the production of leaded gasoline was allowed to continue.

The lead emissions from cars were at their highest levels from 1945 to 1971, and it has been calculated that more than 200 000 tons of lead were emitted on American roads during this period. American children had 300–1000 times higher concentrations of lead in their bodies at that time than they had before leaded gas had been introduced. It was not until 1989 that the U.S. Congress banned leaded gasoline.

Fuller Albright was a young medical student working in Aub's laboratory, who had recently returned to Harvard after having spent a year as a visiting researcher with Jacob Erdheim in Vienna. Albright highly respected Erdheim, whom he thought "knew more about disease processes than anyone else." Albright studied the effects of parathyroid hormone on calcium metabolism, and he was particularly interested in the effects of the hormone on the composition and function of the skeleton. It was logical that the skeleton would be the focus of his studies of calcium regulation since more than 99% of the body's calcium is found in the skeleton and teeth, which means that a parathyroid dysfunction would be expected to lead to skeletal changes.

In 1925, Massachusetts General Hospital opened Ward 4, a clinical research unit specifically equipped for metabolic studies. The ward was one of the first of its kind and it was perfect for physiological studies charting endocrine diseases. The availability of commercial parathyroid preparations had made it possible to study the effects of the hormone in humans. The experimental technique Albright used was based upon studies of patients who had either an excess or deficiency of the hormone. In carefully controlled trials, parathyroid hormone and different electrolytes (calcium and phosphate) were administered in high or low doses after which the resulting effects on the blood, urine and skeleton were studied. These balance studies were complicated and time-consuming, and extreme precision was required when collecting specimens, recording time spans, and performing chemical analyses. No food could be eaten by the patients without its contents determined, every blood sample had to be recorded on the list of losses, and not a single urine sample could be missed. Every day a large number of samples were collected, analyzed, compiled and interpreted – extremely painstaking work. Using this technique, Albright was able to chart the disease mechanisms and hormonal effects in a way no one had ever done before.

Albright found that Martell had a negative calcium balance, in that the calcium losses exceeded the intake, and that the losses were due to an increased resorption of calcium from his skeleton. The team tried to induce a positive calcium balance by giving Martell extra calcium in order to increase its deposition in his calcium-depleted skeleton. This resulted in the calcium levels in his blood going up even higher; the secretion of calcium in his urine increased and new kidney stones developed. They found that Martell's metabolism was similar to that of a healthy person who had been given 100 units of Collip's extract, leading to the conclusion that Martell had an overproduction of parathyroid hormone, that is, he was suffering from an enlarged parathyroid gland. As a consequence, Martell underwent several more neck operations, but to everyone's dismay, no enlarged parathyroids could be found during these operations.

Albright's research was extremely successful and he described, in all, 14 new endocrinological and metabolic disorders or syndromes. He clarified the differences between conditions involving hyperactivity in all of the glands or in single glands, and determined the role of the parathyroids in the formation of kidney stones. He also described new clinical syndromes caused by disorders of the adrenal glands, charted the effect of the sexual hormones and was the first to point out the association between menopause and osteoporosis. His studies also paved the way for the development of birth control pills.

Albright was very careful to protect his time for research, declining every offer from Harvard to make him a professor for fear it would impinge on his research time. The Swedish endocrinologist, Rolf Luft, spent a research period with Albright in the mid-1940s, and when it was time for him to return to Sweden he was advised: "If the Karolinska Institute wants to make you a professor, you should refuse. If you become a professor anyway, then

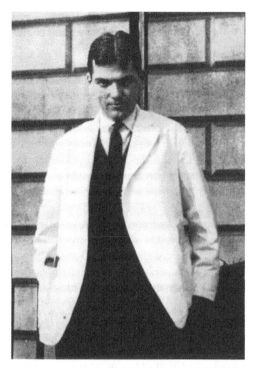

Figure 8.3 Fuller Albright (1900–1969), American endocrinologist working at Massachusetts General Hospital in Boston. Albright laid the foundation for our current understanding of the parathormone's effects. (Used with permission from Lynn Loriaux)

don't become an administrator. If, in spite of everything, you do become a professor and an administrator, then you should in all honesty say goodbye to research." Luft did not follow Albright's advice, instead he became Sweden's first professor of endocrinology and he succeeded in making important discoveries by describing, among other things, a new kind of disorder in the energy-producing structures of the cells (the mitochondria).

Towards the end of the 1920s, more and more patients showed up at Massachusetts General Hospital with a suspected increase in parathyroid activity, but there was no surgeon there with an interest in, or knowledge of, the parathyroids. This was not unexpected as up until then, neck surgery involved steering clear of the small glands in order to avoid precipitating muscle cramps. When the time came to operate on the first patient in Boston, Albright was asked to be present at the operation and to point out the parathyroids for the surgeon as he did not know what they looked like. Albright said later that he felt the earth moving under his feet since he had no idea what parathyroid glands looked like either. The operation was unsuccessful and the surgeon did not find any parathyroid glands. When the next patient was operated on they found a growth "the size of a lemon" of undetermined nature. The subsequent microscopic examination revealed the specimen was conclusively not an enlarged parathyroid gland. After these unsuccessful initial attempts to operate, no more patients were referred to the Harvard surgeons for parathyroid surgery for some time.

The head of the Massachusetts General Surgical Department, Edward Churchill, gave one of his young surgeons, Oliver Cope, the task of studying the anatomy of the parathyroids, the normal microscopic picture and what variations existed regarding the location of the glands. Cope was very thorough, performing neck dissections on 30 autopsy cases. After six months of preparation, Cope operated on two of Albright's patients – both times with successful results. The major challenge, however, was Martell whose condition had continued to deteriorate. The diagnosis hyperparathyroidism seemed clear, but where was the enlarged gland? Martell had undergone three operations in New York and Cope performed three more operations on him – all with negative results. Further attempts seemed futile and, in principle, the surgeons had given up all hope of being able to cure him. Just when Martell's situation seemed hopeless, some new and interesting information unexpectedly came in from across the Atlantic, this time from Stockholm.

On 5th March 1927, a 55-year old woman was admitted to Serafimer Hospital for back pains and marked fatigue. Many examinations were undertaken during her two month stay in the hospital but doctors had been unable to determine the cause of her symptoms, describing her condition in hospital charts as "puzzling." She was discharged with a diagnosis of "neurosis" along with the recommendation to rest up in the countryside.

About two years later, the patient again sought help for her problems, and this time she was admitted to Sabbatsberg Hospital in Stockholm. She had the same complaints as before with headaches, anxiety, heart palpitations, a feeling of pressure on her trachea and oesophagus, weight loss, and fatigue. Many new tests were performed (though none to check the calcium levels in her blood), and most of them produced negative results. A lung X-ray revealed that there was a curved protrusion to the right of the midline in the thorax that went from the upper part of the aortic arch up to the top edge of the breastbone. The abnormality didn't look like either a goitre stretching down into the rib cage, or an aneurysm (a herniated area of a blood vessel). The patient's condition worsened, she became gradually weaker and finally died.

There was a young pathologist named Hilding Bergstrand in the hospital's pathology department who had been made professor of pathology a few years earlier and would later became President of the Karolinska Institute.

For several years Bergstrand had been interested in the pathological changes of the parathyroids and had published several articles on autopsy cases where the parathyroids had been enlarged in combination with changes in other organs, such as the skeleton, the thymus, and the kidneys. During the autopsy of this particular patient Bergstrand found to his great surprise that the growth that had been seen on X-ray consisted of an enlarged parathyroid gland. Thus this parathyroid tumour was located in the chest instead of where it should have been located; in the region of the neck. Microscopic examinations revealed that the patient had von Recklinghausen's disease of the bone and calcifications in the kidneys. Finding a parathyroid gland located inside the thorax was an observation that had been made before, but no one had ever reported evidence that it could be seen on X-ray. This was definitely something worth writing an article about. Bergstrand published a 23-page case study (including X-ray images, photos of the neck organs, and the microscope image) in the *Acta Medica Scandinavica* in December 1931.

Acta Medica Scandinavica was one of 1300 medical periodicals around the world that had its articles indexed according to content in the *Quarterly Cumulative Index Medicus*. The advantage of this well-organised overview was that it allowed researchers to retrieve new articles dealing with a specific field, in this case the parathyroids. *Index Medicus* is no longer published and has been rendered obsolete by the database PubMed, which contains more than 17 million references, abstracts and complete articles from more than 5000 medical journals. It is an invaluable source for all medical researchers and it has open access for everyone.

It did not take long for Fuller Albright and his group to find out about Bergstrand's article. A parathyroid tumour that could be seen on an X-ray – that was exactly the news they needed to hear in Boston. Albright and others on his team had no problems reading the German text and the potential implications for Martell were apparent. Martell soon found out about Bergstrand's article and he insisted that his chest should be explored in an attempt to find the missing parathyroid tumour. To Martell, this possibility of a parathyroid tumour in the chest seemed like his last chance. Many of those around him were skeptical about him undergoing yet another operation. The surgeons were the most hesitant after all the demanding, fruitless operations that had previously been performed, and subjecting Martell to such an extensive and risky surgical procedure did not seem to be a particularly appealing option. Finally, the surgeons Oliver Cope and Edward Churchill conceded and opened Martell's chest. Lo and behold, during this seventh operation a greatly enlarged parathyroid tumour was found. The operation was successful at last. Unfortunately, it turned out to be too late, for Martell died a few weeks later from a kidney infection and renal failure.

The story of Martell's illness was a valuable lesson for all surgeons working with parathyroid surgery: the operations can be technically difficult, repeated operations may sometimes be required and the location of the enlarged gland may vary. Precision and patience are of the essence.

Albright was diagnosed with Parkinson's disease early at 37 years of age. Even though his illness progressed, he continued to be a productive researcher for many years. He decided to try a new method that had not been fully tested in an attempt to lessen his symptoms from the disease. This procedure involved placing a catheter inside the brain, by which an area of the brain could be destroyed by alcohol in a so-called chemical pallidectomy. The technique was in its infancy and its originator, the neurosurgeon Irving Cooper, advised Albright against having the procedure done. Many of his colleagues tried to convince him not to do it, and the dean of Harvard Medical School told him that there were plans to make him a professor and that he therefore ought not to take any risks. Albright answered, "I'd rather be a dead assistant professor than a professor that couldn't function." The procedure was done in June 1956. There was some improvement in the first two days; his shaking lessened and his movements were more precise. On the third day after the operation the catheter that was still in place was removed. Within a few minutes, Albright slipped into a coma caused by cerebral hemorrhage. He never regained consciousness, but he did not die until 1969.

In the beginning of the 1930s, there were many cases of enlarged parathyroids that were successfully treated both in Europe and the United States. The disease hyperparathyroidism had become well established almost half a century after Sandström's discovery of the organ, and his prediction that tumours would be discovered in the organ had proven true. In addition, it had been established that the parathyroid was an organ that was part of the endocrine system, and that hyperparathyroidism was a disease that had chemical, organ-specific, and clinical characteristics. However, the full clinical picture of the disease and its pathophysiological characteristics were far from being completely understood. Although the curative nature of surgery was well established, faulty diagnoses, symptoms related to diseases other than hyperparathyroidism, surgery based on incorrect indications, and unsuccessful operations were not unusual. On the whole, it was still rather unclear as to what kind of disease hyperparathyroidism really was. Could a person have it without having any symptoms? Could symptoms of the disease appear without any changes in the parathyroids? Are there always elevated blood calcium levels in hyperparathyroidism? Does the disease always require an operation? These were the questions that had begun to be asked – indeed, some of them remain unanswered.

Chapter 9 **A disease in disguise**

The early cases of hyperparathyroidism displayed the typical skeletal changes of *osteitis fibrosa cystica*, which made it relatively easy to diagnose the disease by skeletal X-ray and analyzing blood calcium levels. In September 1933 there was an editorial in *The Lancet* that read:

> "Hyperparathyroidism is a conception less than eight years old, and there can be few maladies, old or new, whose mystery has been solved so speedily. A decade ago we had no proof of the relationship between parathyroid activity and the metabolism of phosphorus and calcium, and the advance of knowledge since that time shows medical research at its happiest. The cooperation of medicine, dietetics, experimental pathology, histology, physiology and chemistry has directed the surgeon's knife towards a tumour he could neither see nor feel, and the number of recorded cases of generalised *osteitis fibrosa* which have been arrested or cured by operation is now at least 52. The terrible crippling caused by generalised *osteitis fibrosa* will soon be a thing of the past."

Encouraged by the positive results of parathyroid surgery in the treatment of *osteitis fibrosa cystica*, many parathyroid operations were performed around the world to treat such skeletal diseases as scurvy, "soft bones" or rickets (osteomalacia), and "bamboo spine" (ankylosing spondylitis) – conditions that we now know are not caused by parathyroid disease. The number of patients who were subjected to operations under false pretexts or what complications these operations caused is unknown, but there were many enthusiastic reports about positive effects on these conditions. Reports of cases where there was no improvement were usually avoided. Some orthopaedic surgeons even maintained that parathyroid surgery was an

The Hunt for the Parathyroids, First Edition. Jörgen Nordenström.
© 2013 John Wiley & Sons, Ltd. Published 2013 by John Wiley & Sons, Ltd.

important procedure in the orthopaedic arsenal. During this period of early surgical enthusiasm there were many patients who underwent operations based on faulty indications, for example, elevated calcium levels in the blood due to some cause other than hyperparathyroidism. In other cases, patients were operated on who had normal calcium levels combined with symptoms from the skeleton or joints, while other cases involved psychosocial, mental disorders or general problems – in the absence of parathyroid disorder. Some maintained that there could be a functional overactivity or a 'glandular imbalance' that could be cured by removing one or more of the parathyroids. Others were skeptical as to whether all positive effects could be explained by surgery – although they seemed to have been in the minority.

Today we would classify this as publication bias, meaning that the effect of the procedure was presented as being more successful than it really was because of a selection process in which positive findings are reported more often than negative ones. The results of such a process are deceptive since positive effects of new procedures or treatments may be overestimated and deleterious effects under-reported.

However, even from the earliest operations it was clear that parathyroid surgery was not always an easy task and that it involved many pitfalls. In a candid article with the informative title, "The Vicissitudes of Parathyroid Surgery," Cope described the early experience at Massachusetts General Hospital. Of the first 300 patients who underwent parathyroid surgery, approximately 50 developed complications and had outcomes that were worse than expected. It was obvious that parathyroid surgery could be a technical challenge and it was noted in many cases that the surgeons had been forced to end the operation after a "heart-rending search" in which they had not found the gland or glands which were assumed to be enlarged. In such cases the surgeons were left with an unsolved problem which they did not know how to tackle. Was the missing gland located in the thorax? Should they split the breastbone and search inside the thoracic cavity? Even if four normal glands had been found, was there an additional diseased fifth gland somewhere that they had overlooked?

In many cases the diagnosis was uncertain in spite of extensive investigations, and it was noted that there were other conditions which were similar to hyperparathyroidism. New syndromes were also described. In 30 patients who had originally been thought to be suffering from hyperparathyroidism, it was found that other unrelated disorders were present. Some patients had developed recurrences after previous operations, and some cases were outright surgical failures. Not all patients who had been operated on had elevated calcium levels. Three patients in the series had abnormally low calcium levels, and a new, very unusual disorder was described, pseudohypoparathyroidism. According to Cope, these patients had been operated on because "Dr. Albright wanted to know whether the glands of these patients were suppressed, normal or enlarged" (!).

Several lessons could be learned from these early cases. First, the diagnosis must be correct – hyperparathyroidism was a disorder that could not be diagnosed simply on the basis of the symptoms, and the method used to determine the calcium levels in the blood had to be reliable. The second lesson was that repeated calcium analyses had to be performed as the levels often varied over time; they were sometimes elevated, and sometimes normal. The third lesson had to do with the location of the glands. In three out of four cases the glands were found in typical places, but in the other cases a gland could be hidden within a rather large area. This made identification difficult and greatly complicated the operative procedure. Since it was impossible to know in advance which cases were technically difficult, it was necessary to be focused from the very start of the operation and to avoid all bleeding while dissecting the delicate structures of the neck: the first operation was the golden opportunity to cure the patient.

Cope described these early experiences in terms of "the red ink of parathyroid surgery", but he did not feel that he or his colleagues needed to apologise for their results or for their having followed erroneous indications: "Nothing ventured, nothing gained." Certainly, invaluable new knowledge of parathyroid disease had been gained and several new disorders had been described. In hindsight these early operative results, with an approximately 80% cure rate, must be regarded as rather good considering that chemical methods for determining the concentration of parathyroid hormone were not available, and that enlarged glands could not be radiologically localised. Today it is possible to cure approximately 95% of the patients with hyperparathyroidism with the first operation. This is a result of improved diagnostic methods and localisation studies, but also thanks to the wealth of experience that has been amassed by the pioneers.

Albright's studies during the 1930s suggested that there might be several variants of the disease: one that involved skeletal changes, another that caused kidney stones, and a third variant where the patient had elevated calcium levels but no symptoms from either the skeleton or the kidneys. Many new cases were discovered where the patients exhibited atypical symptoms. The total symptom picture could be diverse and include kidney stones/urinary infections, *osteitis fibrosa cystica*/general osteoporosis, mental/psychosocial problems (fatigue, lack of initiative, depression), muscle fatigue, abdominal problems (ulcers, nausea, loss of appetite), cardiovascular disease and high blood pressure. Patients were even found with undiagnosed hyperparathyroidism who had been locked up in psychiatric wards as a result of incorrect diagnoses. Hyperparathyroidism came to be characterised as a disease comprised of "stones, bones and abdominal groans," with later additions of "psychic moans and fatigue overtones." The clinical symptoms varied as to the kind of complaint and the degree of severity. The only common factor was the elevated calcium levels, but the diagnosis of hyperparathyroidism often remained difficult as many other conditions could also cause increased calcium concentrations.

On 1st July 1969, a new blood analyzing instrument was installed at the Barnes Hospital in St. Louis, Missouri. The instrument, a Technicon SMA 12, was an automated multi-channelled analyser that could simultaneously determine the concentrations of 12 different blood components, including calcium, in a single sample. It was now easy to analyze many different substances, which resulted in the analyzer being used for the blood analysis for all of the patients who sought care in the hospital (actually a kind of biochemical screening). It was soon noted that the number of blood tests with elevated calcium levels increased dramatically, and many new cases of hyperparathyroidism were discovered. During the first 2½ years after the instrument had been installed, 47 patients were operated on for hyperparathyroidism. This was a remarkable increase in the number of performed operations as only 39 patients had undergone surgery during the previous ten years. In these newly discovered cases, there were 12 patients who had no symptoms at all prior to being diagnosed with elevated calcium levels. Eleven other patients were shown, first after surgery, to have had problems related to hyperparathyroidism, and the remaining 24 patients had been admitted for operations with classic symptoms of hyperparathyroidism. Consequently, about 50% of the patients that had been discovered by biochemical screening were asymptomatic when the elevated calcium levels were discovered in their blood.

Thus this biochemical screening procedure resulted in many new cases of hyperparathyroidism being discovered as a result of serendipity – a fortunate, unexpected discovery. The term serendipity was coined in the mid-1700s by the Earl of Oxford, Horace Walpole, to denote a chance discovery of something valuable that occurs when one is occupied with some other activity – in other words intellectually taking advantage of an unexpected discovery or observation, in contrast to a more structured search. Walpole took the word serendipity from the Persian fairytale, "The Three Princes of Serendip," in *The Book of One Thousand and One Nights*. In this tale the princes repeatedly discovered valuable things which they could make great use of, but which they had not been looking for, and used them to escape difficult situations.

Randall and Keating used the term serendipity to connote the cases of hyperparathyroidism that were discovered by chance during a biochemical screening. There are many other examples of serendipities in the history of medicine, such as Wilhelm Röntgen's discovery of X-rays, Becquerel's finding of natural radioactivity and John Cade's discovery of lithium as a treatment for bipolar psychiatric disorders. Perhaps the most famous example is Alexander Fleming's discovery of penicillin.

Similar patterns to those that had been discovered at the Barnes Hospital were observed at other hospitals using automated blood analyzers. This resulted in a dramatic increase in the number of individuals diagnosed with elevated calcium levels due to hyperparathyroidism. From having previously been an unusual disease with clear symptoms, the clinical picture changed and hyperparathyroidism became a relatively common disease with a mild clinical presentation. Population studies showed that hyperparathyroidism could be found in one or two out of every 1000 people (0.1–0.2%). The disease was found to be about three times more prevalent in women than in men, and was especially common in women over 45–50 years of age. Approximately 20–30 out of every 1000 women (2–3%) could be shown to have the disease. Also remarkable was the fact that approximately half of these patients who were discovered by biochemical screening had only slightly elevated calcium levels, no particular symptoms, and no skeletal disease or kidney stone disorders either. A new disease entity had been discovered: "biochemical" or "asymptomatic" hyperparathyroidism. The number of cases classified as asymptomatic varied between the different centres. Considerable debate existed and some endocrinologists maintained that 80% of their patients had no symptoms while others thought that very few of their patients could be considered to be completely symptom-free. A common estimate was that approximately half of the patients could be considered asymptomatic, or had only mild signs of hyperparathyroidism.

As a result, the clinical picture changed noticeably after 1960 compared to 1930–1960. During the earlier period the patients had more specific and serious symptoms involving the skeleton, kidney stones, higher calcium levels, and lower phosphate levels indicative of a higher hormonal activity. The patients were also younger and the parathyroid tumours were larger during the earlier period.

The many new cases of hyperparathyroidism discovered through biochemical screening, resulted in operations for this new variant of the disease becoming common at most major hospitals throughout the Western world. Some endocrinologists, who had observed patients with asymptomatic hyperparathyroidism who had not been operated on, found that this did not result in any apparent disadvantages to them: their calcium levels remained mildly elevated and few patients developed complications from their disease. It therefore seemed that the asymptomatic variant was perhaps not an early stage of the classic form of hyperparathyroidism. Perhaps it could be a more benign form of the disease? It began to be questioned whether every patient diagnosed with hyperparathyroidism really needed an operation. Most of them had no symptoms at all; their slightly elevated blood calcium values remained stable and complications did not seem to develop. Furthermore many of these elderly women in their 70s were somewhat hesitant about undergoing an operation when no clear advantage could be expected as a result. They felt healthy, so how could they become healthier by having neck surgery?

The problem of knowing what to do with all these patients with asymptomatic hyperparathyroidism brought up the perpetual question of what a disease is and when can a person be considered healthy? Some attempts to define the concept of 'disease' focus on an impaired ability to function, for example "a state of impaired health or a condition that causes abnormal function", or "a disease is a bodily or mental state that leads to an impaired function or discomfort for the affected individual." Other attempts to define disease use its opposite, health. One such well-known definition is the one stated by WHO: "Health is a state of complete physical, mental and social well-being and not merely the absence of disease or infirmity." The problem with WHO's definition is that, in reality, it results in most people being considered unhealthy. Both disease and health are concepts that are very vague and difficult to define. The epidemiologist Geoffrey Rose maintains: "There is no disease that you either have or don't have – except perhaps sudden death and rabies. All other diseases you either have a little or a lot of." Ivan Illich stressed the social dimensions of the concept of health and disease: "Each civilization defines its own diseases. What is sickness in one might be a chromosomal abnormality, a crime, a divinity or a sin in another." Illich has repeatedly warned about the consequences of widespread medicalisation of society.

The story *The Last Well Person* by N.M. Hadler is about a 53-year-old mathematics teacher in the American Midwest who caused a sensation in the medical establishment when it was shown that nothing could be found wrong with him in spite of extensive testing. However he was the only known person in the entire world who was lacking any sign of a medical deviation.

When doctors are asked what can be considered a disease, their answers often stress that it must be possible to diagnose the condition and that a treatment should exist. Sometimes it is suggested half jokingly that, "a healthy person is a person that hasn't been thoroughly examined." Is a person healthy when all of the medical examinations and blood tests show values that fall within the so-called normal range? And what is a normal range? As a rule, one does not refer to a normal range but rather to a reference range which is established by testing a large group of seemingly healthy individuals and determining the reference range; for example, as ± 2 standard deviations from the established mean for the particular test in the particular population. This means that 2.5% of the individuals in the group are going to have a value that is lower than the lowest value in the reference range and just as many will have a value that is higher than the highest value in the reference range. As a result, 5% of the individuals, or about every 20th individual, will have values that lie outside of the reference range even though they may not necessarily be sick. In reality this also means that if 20 different blood analyses are performed, statistically speaking one of these will lie outside of the established reference interval – even though this particular individual may not be sick. Thus it cannot be assumed that an individual is sick simply because of a deviating value; the signs of the disease that are usually linked to the measured deviation must also be found.

What then are the criteria that have to be met for a disease to exist? Surveys have been made among healthy people and healthcare workers who were given a list of different conditions and asked to note which criteria they felt needed to be met for a disease to exist. Diseases such as malaria, tuberculosis, cancer, diabetes, asthma, all end up at the top of the list in these kinds of surveys. Far down the list are conditions like red-green colour-blindness, nearsightedness, tennis elbow, hangover, heatstroke and old age.

Tuberculosis meets many of the criteria that would class it as a disease. The infection can be linked to a specific bacterium, there are characteristic symptoms and there are drugs that can eliminate the bacteria, after which the sick person recovers. Koch isolated tubercle bacteria in 1884 and effective treatments have been available since the 1940s. However tuberculosis has existed for thousands of years – which shows that the requirements that the bacteria can be isolated and that the disease can be treated are not essential requirements for a disease to exist.

Is heart disease a disease? A heart attack is certainly an illness that is usually caused by arteriosclerotic constrictions in the heart's coronary arteries. Yet arteriosclerotic changes begin early in life, and most individuals have more or less marked changes in their coronary arteries as they age. Can one really speak of "heart disease" when 100% of a certain age group has arteriosclerotic changes in the heart's coronary artery?

Campbell maintains in *The Concept of Disease* that the characteristic features of conditions that can be classed as diseases are, first, that they are linked to an abnormal structure or function (they have an underlying cause) and, secondly, that the condition is usually treated by a doctor. Without doctors there can be no patients. Problems arise in this medical discourse when discussing conditions where the cause is unknown and where no specific diagnostic instruments or no effective treatments exist. Conditions like electrical allergies, oral galvanism, chronic fatigue syndrome and burnout are diagnoses or concepts that are difficult for medicine to deal with, and the number of individuals who are sick tends to vary over time without there being any obvious explanation.

Several years ago the *British Medical Journal* encouraged their readers to nominate conditions that could be called "non-diseases." They received many suggestions such as pregnancy, hangover, jet lag, grey hair, freckles and old age. An intense discussion followed and some readers felt that the entire argument was absurd. The editor maintained that the study had served its purpose: the concepts of disease, non-disease and health are difficult to define, and there is no consensus as to their meaning.

After some time it became clear that hyperparathyroidism was a disease that could appear in many different guises. The concept of "asymptomatic hyperparathyroidism" was particularly problematic since there were no firm scientific data that could be used to determine whether the condition should be treated or not. Many endocrinologists felt that it might not be necessary to operate on all patients diagnosed with hyperparathyroidism, and that it might be more reasonable to follow the development and operate on cases that worsened or where complications threatened to arise. Surgeons were generally more inclined to treat a disease with a relatively straight forward operation when the alternative would involve years of checkups in physicians' offices.

Different routines were developed in different places and the attitude towards surgical intervention varied from doctor to doctor. The need for some kind of consensus on asymptomatic hyperparathyroidism became more obvious, and in 1990 a group of leading doctors and researchers in the field met to draw up recommendations. There was general agreement that patients who had clear symptoms or had developed complications of the disease (e.g. fractures or kidney stones) should be offered surgery. An operation should also be recommended to patients with markedly elevated calcium levels (higher than 2.85 millimoles per litre), elevated levels of calcium secretion in the urine, impaired kidney function, or with osteoporosis. In addition, it was felt that relatively young patients (under 50 years of age) and patients who could not get regular checkups should be offered surgery. Patients who did not meet these criteria could be categorised as having a mild or an asymptomatic form of the disease, and it was felt that they could be monitored to ensure that they did not develop complications.

At later follow-up meetings it was felt that the prior recommendations, with a few minor adjustments, should continue to be valid. As is often the case when "consensus" is involved, there were those who disagreed, which meant variable adherence to the guidelines. The majority of patients are probably cared for according to these recommendations, but some patients do not want to endure living with a disease if it can be cured, and some doctors maintain that the disadvantages, including the need for repeated checkups, outweigh the advantages recommending surgical management as soon as a diagnosis has been made.

Christmas Eve, 1989. The patient M. S., who was almost unconscious, was admitted to a hospital in Stockholm. She was 65 years old, and for many years she had been treated with lithium for manic-depressive psychosis. A blood test taken on arrival showed a calcium level of 5.07 millimoles per litre (100% higher than the high end of the reference range), close to life-threatening. The patient was having a so-called calcium crisis which was caused by severe hyperparathyroidism. That this condition is particularly dramatic is evident from the different names given to it: parathyroid poisoning, acute hyperparathyroidism, hypercalcaemic crisis and hyper-hyperparathyroidism Her acute critical condition was treated with abundant hydration and calcitonin (a hormone that lowers blood calcium levels) and she was operated on a few days later. A parathyroid gland that was more than 100 times larger than normal (about 5 grams) was found, along with two more slightly enlarged parathyroids. The patient recovered from the operation and could return home soon afterwards. She had suffered an episode of lithium-induced hyperparathyroidism.

In the beginning of the 1970s it was reported that patients who were being treated with lithium for manic-depressive psychoses could be affected by unexpected complications, one of which was elevated calcium levels caused by hyperparathyroidism. Lithium is chemical element number 3 in the periodic system and belongs to the group of alkali metals. It was discovered by Johan August Arfwedson in 1817 in a piece of mineral taken from a mine on the island of Utö in Stockholm's archipelago. Lithium is a common element and soon became a popular patent medicine for treating gout, indigestion, and gall stones. The St. Louis businessman, Charles Leiper Gripp, developed a citrus flavoured soft drink that contained lithium. It was first called Bib-Label Lithiated Lemon Lime Soda – a complicated name that was later changed to *7-Up*. Lithium was removed from the product in 1950 when it was reported that its substitution for ordinary table salt could cause heart problems.

In the 1940s, Australian psychiatrist John Cade discovered that lithium was effective for the treatment of bipolar disorders and it has since then been shown to be one of neuropharmacology's most effective drugs. As has often been the case in medicine, Cade's discovery was a chance happening – a serendipity. Cade speculated that there could be similar mechanisms involved in manic-depressive illness and thyroid disorders comparing manic episodes to hyperthyroidism and depressive episodes to hypofunction. Cade concentrated his efforts on trying to identify a substance that was in surplus during the manic episodes and scarce during depressive episodes. After having completed a number of animal experiments, he began to suspect that urea contributed to the different manifestations of bipolar disorders. There was, however, one problem with Cade's hypothesis: the level of urea in the patients' urine did not seem to be any higher during the manic phase than during the depressive phase. This did not deter Cade and he continued with new experiments. When he tested different preparations on laboratory animals he had problems with the relatively insoluble uric acid. The answer to this problem was to use lithium urate which is the most soluble of the urate salts. To his surprise, he found that the animals did not become more active when they were given a more concentrated solution; instead, they became calmer and sometimes even apathetic. He was later able to show that the effect was related to the lithium and not to the uric acid, as he had originally thought.

Cade tested lithium on a small group of psychiatric patients and found that those with manic-depressive psychosis responded especially well: both the manic and the depressive episodes were milder. Yet, problems arose despite the promising results of his early experiments. High doses of lithium caused serious side effects and there were even deaths as a result of lithium poisoning. Gradually chemical methods were developed that could determine the lithium concentration in the blood, making it possible to determine a therapeutic interval that made the treatment safer. Another problem lay in the fact that lithium was an element with no patent potential leading to a lack of interest from the pharmaceutical industry. After years of experiments, lithium became firmly established as a cornerstone in the treatment of bipolar disorders and Cade finally received the recognition he deserved. Cade remained humble about his chance discovery, describing himself as merely a gold prospector who happened to find a nugget.

Long-term treatment of manic-depressive illness with lithium often has a mild effect on the calcium and parathyroid hormone levels of these patients, but sometimes hyperparathyroidism can develop. This may require surgical management in some cases.

Chapter 10 **The elusive hormone**

The parathyroid extracts developed by Collip and Hanson were used in numerous animal experiments and experimental clinical studies, leading to significant advances in the understanding of the function of the parathyroid hormone. The extract could be used to correct a parathyroid hypofunction or to study the effects of excessive dosages, but the results were often difficult to interpret. Sometimes similar results could not be obtained even if the experiments were repeated under identical conditions. Different preparations gave dissimilar results, and different ways of administering the hormone gave varying results in different organ systems. Some researchers maintained that there were a number of active components in the extract that had different effects on calcium and phosphate metabolism as well as on the kidneys and blood pressure regulation. It was unclear whether these different effects were caused by the actual physiological effects of the hormone or whether they were due to impurity of the extract.

The frustration over the failure to produce pure parathyroid hormone was noted in a report from the early 1950s where it was concluded that either the active substance of the parathyroid consisted of a very large protein that broke down during the isolation process into a number of different biologically active fractions, or the active component was not a large protein at all. Perhaps it was a small molecule that was bound to different substances in the extract? Thus it seemed impossible to chemically characterise a hormone that split up into a number of smaller parts or gave rise to new constellations during the extraction process.

A puzzle or a mystery? Gregory Treverton, an American security analyst, has emphasised the importance of making a distinction between these notions in order to solve problems. According to Treverton, a puzzle is a situation where one does not have enough information on hand to solve

The Hunt for the Parathyroids, First Edition. Jörgen Nordenström.
© 2013 John Wiley & Sons, Ltd. Published 2013 by John Wiley & Sons, Ltd.

the problem. There are pieces missing preventing the puzzle from being solved, and one small detail can sometimes be crucial. A mystery, on the other hand, is a situation where all of the necessary information is available and where there is too much (often irrelevant) information instead of too little. Judgment, experience and special skills are needed to solve a mystery – one must understand the information that exists and interpret it correctly. As an example, Treverton used the problem of knowing where to find Osama Bin-Laden. This was, for a long time, a puzzle since it could easily have been solved, for example by someone in Bin-Laden's closest circle revealing his location. On the other hand, the complex situation in Iraq was considered to be a mystery, since the problem had economic, social, political, cultural and historical causes and no single piece of the puzzle could be expected to solve it. Mysteries are more common than puzzles in the social and economic sciences. In the natural sciences puzzles are more frequent than mysteries. The Nobel Prizes in the sciences are awarded to people who have solved puzzles, not those who have solved mysteries.

It was not until 35 years after Collip's and Hanson's extracts had been developed that the hormone could successfully be isolated and the chemical structure determined. After decades of frustrating attempts, it was finally realised that the method of tissue extraction using warm hydrochloric acid released the hormone and made it soluble, but also caused the hormone's long chain of amino acids to split at different sites during the process. This led to the generation of fragments of different lengths with different biological activities. Some fragments exhibited nearly the same activity as the complete hormone, others were inactive, and still other fragments even had opposite (calcium lowering) effects. By abandoning the hydrochloric acid method and using organic solvents instead, Auerbach was able to isolate the hormone in its entirety in 1959. This breakthrough soon made it possible to determine the chemical composition of parathyroid hormone and to produce it synthetically. It was discovered that the intact hormone consisted of a long chain containing 84 amino acids. By using the knowledge that warm hydrochloric acid splits the hormone into fragments, researchers were able to show that the biological activity of the hormone was linked to the first 34 amino acids. Surprisingly enough, it was discovered that the biological activity of the 34-amino-acid fragment was identical to that of the complete 84-amino-acid-long hormone.

To measure is to know, according to the 19th century physicist Lord Kelvin. The possibility of diagnosing and thereby understanding the diseases of the parathyroids and other endocrine glands was limited for a long time because there were no methods available for determining the concentration of different hormones in the blood; this meant that some patients, with elevated concentrations of calcium in their blood, were operated on in the belief that they had a parathyroid disorder, when they actually had elevated calcium levels for other reasons. The reason for the methodological difficulties in determining the hormone concentrations in the blood was that the amounts of hormones circulating within the blood are very low. Some hormones are found in concentrations as low as one trillionth of one gram (a picogram) per decilitre of blood.

The lack of methods to determine the blood concentrations of different hormones made it impossible to diagnose many endocrine diseases until later phases, after clear signs of illness or complications had appeared. Some endocrine diseases are caused by hormone deficiencies, others by a surplus, a dysfunctional effect or a change in the metabolism of the hormone. In most cases it was impossible to determine which one of these was the actual cause. The entire field of endocrinology was in danger of hitting a dead end due to lack of reliable methods for determining the concentration of different hormones in the blood.

Rosalyn Yalow and Solomon Berson succeeded in developing a method for determining hormone levels in the blood. It was based on the application of radioactive antibodies to hormones. The description of their method in the *Journal of Clinical Investigation* in 1960 marked a breakthrough in endocrinological research, and it is one of the most cited medical texts. A search of "radioimmunoassay" in the medical database PubMed returns more than 85 000 results, and a search on Google returns more than four million results. Yalow was awarded the Nobel Prize in 1977 for this discovery. Berson had died a few years earlier and could not be awarded the prize posthumously.

The method that Yalow and Berson developed, radioimmunoassay (RIA), was as ingenious it was simple. The method is based on the use of two antibodies. The first antibody is mixed with a hormone that has been labelled with a radioactive agent so that an antigen-antibody complex is formed. Blood containing an unknown concentration of the hormone is then added to the solution. In this mixture, the unlabelled hormone will compete with the radiolabelled hormone for the binding sites of the antibody. The more of the unlabelled hormone present in the sample, the less radioactive hormone is bound. A second antibody is added to separate bound antigen from free antigen. The radioactivity in fractions of bound and free antigens, respectively, are then compared with a standard curve with the same procedure done with known concentrations of the hormone.

The way the method works can be illustrated by the game musical chairs: We mix antibodies (= chairs), labelled hormone molecules (= children with hats), and a small volume of patient's plasma (= children without hats). We can only see children playing the game if they are wearing hats

(= radiolabelled hormone molecules). If we have many children without hats in the game (= a high hormone concentration in the patient's blood), then when the music stops many children with hats (= radiolabelled hormone molecules) will fail to find a chair (= an antibody). From the ratio of children without hats to children with hats, it is possible to calculate the number of children without hats (i.e. the hormone concentration in the blood sample).

The most remarkable characteristic of the RIA method is its incredible sensitivity. It can measure inconceivably low concentrations of almost every kind of substance. Antibodies can find, bind, and make it possible to determine a hormone among a myriad of substances that can be found in concentrations that are several million times greater in the same blood sample. The method has sensitivity comparable to the possibility of determining the sugar content of a lake that is 100 kilometres long by 100 kilometres wide by 10 metres deep after pouring 1 tablespoon of granulated sugar into the water!

In order to avoid working with radioactive materials, another method is now used; the Enzyme-Linked ImmunoSorbent Assay (ELISA) by which colour changes (fluorescence) are analyzed instead of radioactivity, but the principle is the same. RIA was truly a breakthrough.

Considering the initial conditions, the road to success was long and in no way self-evident. If we go back to 1950 when Yalow and Berson began their collaboration, the conditions were as follows:

- a small radioisotope department at the Bronx Veterans Administration Hospital in New York that did not consist of much more than a lab bench and equipment for measuring radioactivity;
- Rosalyn Yalow, a 29-year-old nuclear physicist with no formal training in either biology or medicine;
- Solomon Berson, a 32-year-old newly licensed internist with almost no research experience;
- minimal funding from the hospital's internal medical department to start research using radioactive isotopes.

Under these conditions, certainly no one could have possibly imagined that the research results to be produced during the following 20 years would ever lead to a Nobel Prize in Medicine.

Rosalyn Yalow had received her Ph.D. degree in nuclear physics at the University of Illinois. She was admitted to the doctoral program in 1941 as the only woman. They admitted a woman in order to ensure that a student place did not go unfilled as so many young men had been drafted into military service during World War II. She was accepted on the stipulation that she "would not become a burden on the university" after she graduated. At that time Yalow was the lone woman in a faculty of 400 people and she commented on this later by saying, "they had to start a war to get a woman in the department." She finished her studies in record time with the highest grades and then moved to New York and began working part-time as a nuclear physicist and part-time as a medical secretary in the newly established Radiophysics Department of the Bronx VA Hospital.

Solomon Berson has been described as multi-talented: gifted in mathematics, a good violinist, and a master class chess and bridge player – a true Renaissance figure. Berson had applied to study medicine at 21 different medical schools before finally being admitted to New York University Medical School where he graduated with top honours. One wonders what the entrance requirements were for the 20 universities that turned Berson down since they were unable to identify a person who would later be one of the best students and an exceptionally successful medical doctor and researcher.

Yalow and Berson began studying the problem of measuring the blood volume of the body as their first project. They continued with studies on iodine and thyroid function, albumin, and later insulin and other hormones. They soon had their first publication in *Science* dealing with how the blood volume could be determined with the aid of radioactive potassium. This was truly a remarkable achievement, but the major breakthrough came several years later with their studies on insulin and the development of the RIA method.

Eugene Strauss, one of Yalow and Berson's colleagues, described in his book, *Rosalyn Yalow - Her Life and Work in Medicine*, the atmosphere and the activity in the little isotope department in the Bronx that was soon to become highly respected and widely known. The department performed both medical radioisotope diagnostics and research. The money earned doing routine analyses for clinical work paid for their research. This meant Yalow and Berson never had to apply for any research funding.

The RIA method could have been a source of large royalty revenues for Yalow and Berson, but they never patented their method. They wanted the method to be freely available for use in the research community and in medicine. A sympathetic point of view, but also somewhat naive, since many pharmaceutical companies have made large profits from the commercialisation of the method. Surely RIA would not have been particularly more expensive or less available if Yalow and Berson, or their institution, had been paid royalties for the commercialisation of the technique. Yalow commented that they did not apply for a patent because they "did not have time for such things."

The decision not to patent the RIA method had perhaps been influenced by the fact that the Curies had declined patenting their method for producing radium. Pierre and Marie ceded their rights to the production method even though they were well aware that a patent would probably generate high revenues and prosperity, including a first-class laboratory.

Eve Curie described the discussion about the patent issue as a five-minute conversation in which Marie completely rejected the thought of applying for a patent:

> "It is customary among us physicists that we publish our research results with no restrictions. It is mostly a matter of pure chance whether our discovery will be shown to have industrial and commercial prospects in the future. We cannot take advantage of this, and besides, our radium will be used as a medicine to treat a disease. I cannot see why we should receive any personal gain from our discovery. That would contradict the spirit of science."

In 1963, Berson, Yalow, Auerbach and Potts described an RIA method for determining parathyroid hormone. For the first time, it was now possible to measure the parathyroid hormone levels in the blood, and it was found that patients with hyperparathyroidism had higher levels in their blood than individuals with no known parathyroid disease. However, the new method for analyzing parathyroid hormone levels was soon fraught with problems. As it turned out, it was the most difficult of many RIA methods. The immunisation process that Berson and Yalow used created different antibodies which, when bound to the hormone, were shown to disappear from the bloodstream at varying rates. It was also found that the parathyroid hormone that existed in the blood and the hormone that could be extracted from diseased glands each had different immunological characteristics. The reasons for these conflicting observations were shown to have been caused by the antibodies binding to different fragments of the hormone. Once again the old problem of different size fragments of the complete hormone had not been solved. The limitations of the method were so great that in many cases it was not possible to separate with certainty the patients who had hyperparathyroidism from those who had not simply by using parathyroid hormone and calcium analyses.

In 1968 Berson received a professorship in medicine at the Mount Sinai School of Medicine. Some time after Berson became a professor, one of his older professor colleagues asked:

> "How many papers have you published, Sol?"
> "I'm ashamed to say that I have published more than one hundred papers," Berson responded.
> "I've published 384 papers," said the colleague.
> "Well," Berson answered, "I said that I was ashamed of the number of publications, but the reason is that I haven't made a hundred significant discoveries. . . . How many have you made?"

For a very long time attempts have been made to measure scientific quality by using bibliometric methods. Just listing the number of published articles obviously does not signify the scientific quality of the work. It is comparable to little boys trying to measure their manhood in centimetres or inches. One method that is often used to measure "scientific weight" is to evaluate the so-called impact factor of an article. This assessment is based on the fact that researchers prefer to publish their work in periodicals that are very prestigious and these publications have a large number of manuscripts submitted for review. This means that the editors of the highest rated periodicals can pick and choose among the articles they consider to be particularly important, maybe even epoch-making. The impact factor is measured according to the number of citations for an article in a particular periodical that appear in other publications. Today there are more than 5000 medical periodicals and 75% of them have an impact factor that is lower than two. The periodicals that have very high impact factors include *Nature, Science,* the *New England Journal of Medicine,* the *Journal of Clinical Investigation* – publications in which Berson and Yalow had their work published several times.

Many researchers are critical of the entire concept of an impact factor because the classification is based on the periodical's quality or ranking rather than the importance or the quality of the article. The publications with the highest impact factors almost exclusively contain articles dealing with basic scientific discoveries in molecular biology or chemistry, for example, and very seldom observations or discoveries having more immediate implications for medicine and health care. Many clinicians at university hospitals therefore feel that they are treated unfairly by the system – especially when the university's research funding is based on these kinds of evaluations. Just how this kind of numerical exercise can be translated into better health, less mortality or better medical care is unclear.

Another standard often used to measure scientific quality is citation frequency, that is, the number of times that a work has been quoted by other researchers. Methodological descriptions (the RIA method is a good example here) usually have the highest citation frequency for the simple reason that all articles have to precisely describe the method that was used. Measuring scientific production and quality is therefore difficult, and it is noteworthy that some researchers, who place much weight on the use of good methodology and critical thinking within their own scientific discipline, are so uncritical and unscientific when it comes to direct comparisons between different researchers or research teams. In some respects it is easier to identify a good researcher when you meet one than to define one by using bibliometric methods.

Berson was highly respected by his colleagues at the clinic, but he was soon on a collision course with the hospital's administration which did not share his vision of academic medicine. The hospital board wanted to run the hospital as an effective health care institution, while Berson felt that the medical care given at a university hospital could only be justified if it could support medical research and education. For Berson, this led to a bitter struggle to safeguard the academic part of the hospital's programme. Berson had to bicker with the hospital administration about rooms for research and teaching, the number of beds that could be used for medical care and teaching and the number of staff positions in the department. This struggle for academic quality would prove to be futile and Berson became increasingly disillusioned about the developments at the hospital. A new time had come where professional healthcare administrators, often with backgrounds as medical practitioners, set the agenda for the hospital's development. On Friday, 9th April 1972 the director of the hospital marched into Berson's office and informed him that he had been relieved of his position as head of the clinic. Berson left New York the same day to participate in a scientific conference in Atlantic City. On Sunday he was found dead in his hotel room after having suffered a heart attack.

One of Yalow's earliest role models had been Marie Curie, and she felt that every future woman researcher should read Ève Curie's book, *Madame Curie – A Biography*. In an article in the *New York Times Magazine* in 1978, Yalow was described as "a Madame Curie from the Bronx" – a fitting description since their careers exhibited many similarities. They were both physicists who worked with radioactivity and both had succeeded in combining exceptional careers with their roles as mothers and wives. When Yalow was awarded the Nobel Prize in Medicine, only the second woman to ever receive one, she naturally became an example for women researchers and her successes made research done by women more respected.

Only in 1970, almost one hundred years after Sandström had discovered the parathyroid glands, was it possible to establish the exact chemical structure of the parathyroid hormone. When this had finally been accomplished, the hormone could be produced synthetically, thus avoiding having to extract it from animal tissue. The effects of the intact hormone, as well as the different fragments of the hormone, could now be studied. It was established that this was a hormone that was unusually unstable, and that certain parts of the intact hormone would split into pieces after it had been secreted into the bloodstream. This was reflected in the occurrence of a number of different fragments having different biological activities. Also the relative number of different fragments varied widely in both hyperfunction and hypofunction of the parathyroids. This explained why hormone analyses using antibodies aimed at different parts of the hormone showed different results when there was an abnormal function of the organ.

Ever since Felix Mandl's operation on the first case of hyperparathyroidism, surgeons had been looking for a method that would make it possible to exactly localise a diseased enlarged parathyroid gland. Hilding Bergstrand's case report from 1931, in which an X-ray showed an enlarged parathyroid inside the thorax, had unfortunately turned out to be a rare exception. Ernest Lawrence developed the cyclotron in 1931. This paved the way for Irène Curie, Marie's and Pierre's elder daughter, and her husband Frédéric Joliot, who were later successful in producing artificial isotopes. The first isotope was radioactive aluminium which was produced by using polonium irradiation. As a young girl, Irène had seen her mother receive the Nobel Prize in Chemistry from the Swedish King Gustaf V, and 24 years later she and her husband received their own Nobel Prizes in Chemistry presented by the same monarch. The new artificial radioactivity that had been created by the Joliots very quickly gave rise to a number of different applications in medicine: as a method to treat leukaemia and hyperthyroidism, as a trace element for studying the metabolism of different organic and inorganic substances (including calcium), and for determining the function of different organs (e.g. the thyroid gland).

During the 1970s, isotopes were developed that made it possible to visualise most organs in the body. Even though it was sometimes possible to confirm an enlarged parathyroid gland with the aid of radioactive caesium, thallium or technetium, the examinations using these isotopes were not very reliable. The frustration over the unreliable localisation methods was well summarised by the American radiologist John Doppman, who maintained, "The only localisation method that a patient with hyperparathyroidism needs is to localise an experienced parathyroid surgeon." A few years later it was shown that a radiopharmaceutical that had been developed for examining the heart muscle, technetium-99-sestamibi, could reveal enlarged parathyroids in patients with hyperparathyroidism better than previously used agents. Sestamibi-exams were not completely reliable, but they were at least sensitive enough to help diagnose an overactive gland in most cases, and could thus help the surgeon pinpoint the problem. Ultrasound proved to have reliability similar to that of sestamibi, and if both of these methods were combined, the reliability was even greater. These localisation techniques paved the way for more directed and less extensive surgical procedures.

Every surgeon remembers the occasion of, or at least the feelings associated with, their first skin incision during their first operation. Making the first skin incision did not only mean that you opened a door to an inner structure, it also meant that you had been allowed to enter the circle of surgeons and the world of surgery. Since time immemorial the actual skin incision has been an almost ritual act that has linked together the surgeon with the patient and surgeons

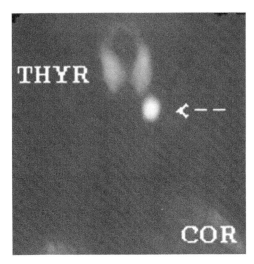

Figure 10.1 Sestamibi scintigraphy. The arrow depicts an increased isotope uptake in an enlarged parathyroid gland. Isotope uptake is also found in the two thyroid lobes (THYR) and in the heart (COR). (Used with permission from Hans Jacobsson MD, PhD)

with other surgeons. Many operations can be performed by making small incisions, but sometimes incisions must be made that are some 30 cm long, for example from the breastbone down to the pubic bone. "Big incisions – big operations – big surgeons." Many surgeons have had their names inscribed in the history of surgery because of their skin incisions, including Kocher for his neck incision for goitre surgery, McBurney for appendix operations and Pfannenstiel for uterine operations. Imagining an operation with no scalpel or skin incision was impossible for most people prior to the mid-1980s.

The surgical paradigm that large operations required large incisions gave way in 1985 when the German surgeon Erich Mühe succeeded in removing a gall bladder by using a laparoscope and an insertion instrument made out of a bicycle handlebar instead of making a conventional skin incision. Mühe was initially met with skepticism when he presented his method at the different German surgical conferences, and his first reports were rejected by a number of periodicals. Some felt that Mühe's technique was "Mickey Mouse surgery," if not downright dangerous: "small incisions – small brains." Eventually the method was adopted by French and American surgeons, and this was the start of laparoscopic surgery. After some time Mühe received the recognition he was due, and the method quickly spread around the world. The technique was used for procedures that previously required large skin incisions: operations on the stomach, the large intestine, the adrenal glands, the lungs, and the heart. The scalpel disappeared as a symbol of surgery. One would have thought that the development would have ended here with the ability to perform major procedures through a few small holes in the abdominal wall that needed little suturing. Yet the boundaries for how far this development could progress did not stop. Nowadays, many advanced procedures can be performed by using catheters that are inserted through blood vessels in the groin, including ruptured aortic aneurysms and defective leaks between the two chambers of the heart. It is even possible to remove an appendix by means of an endoscope inserted through the mouth – an abdominal operation with no external scar.

Developments in laparoscopy opened the way for computer-assisted procedures (robotic surgery) in which a light source, camera and a surgical instrument are inserted into the area to be operated on. In robotic surgery the surgeon sits a few metres away from the patient so that he or she can steer the instruments via a control panel with the aid of a two or three-dimensional image. In September 2001, "Operation Lindberg" was performed. This time it had nothing to do with a solo flight across the Atlantic. Instead it was telesurgery with the surgeon in New York and the patient lying on an operating table in the Hôpital Civil in Strasbourg. An entire staff of telecommunication technicians and computer experts assisted the operating personnel. By using high-speed fibre optics and robotic techniques, the surgeon in New York could navigate the instruments with precision inside the abdomen of a 68-year old woman and perform a gallstone operation 7000 km away. One of the problems that had to be solved was time delay. A time delay of more than half a second would have been dangerous, but the time delay was reduced to 80 milliseconds.

Today robotic surgery has become a standard operating procedure for early cases of prostate cancer and other applications are being developed.

The improved possibilities of localising a diseased enlarged parathyroid gland with the aid of sestamibi has made it possible to perform more precise and directed parathyroid operations. The concept of minimally invasive surgery was also developed for the parathyroids and it came to include centimetre-long skin incisions, walk-in surgery, operations using local anaesthesia and endoscopy with the aid of a video camera. In a sense, parathyroid surgery had come full circle: from Felix Mandl's operation using local anaesthesia in 1925 to minimally invasive surgery 70 years later. The difference today is that we often know where the enlarged gland is located, and by measuring the parathyroid hormone levels during an operation, it is possible to confirm that the over-productive gland has been removed. Today parathyroid operations are no longer the hazardous procedures that they used to be thanks to better localisation methods, and most patients can be cured by a single operation.

Chapter 11 **The language of god**

A monastery garden is an unlikely place to start a revolution, but this is exactly where Gregor Mendel laid the foundation for genetics. In studies that were done over several years around 1860, Mendel used the garden pea plant, *pisum sativum*, to study the heredity pattern of seven different traits: the colour and shape of the ripe pea (grey and smooth, or white and wrinkled), the colour of the cotyledon (yellow or green), the shape of the ripe pods (full or constricted), the colour of the unripe pods (green or yellow), the colour of the flowers (white or purple), the position of the flowers (terminal – at the top, or axial – along the stem), the length of the stem (long or short). The predominant theory at that time was that heredity constituted a kind of "hereditary mix" whereby offspring would be something of an average mixture of the parents' traits. Mendel found, however, that the hybrid progeny did not exhibit a mixture of the parents' characteristics, but rather that they were identical to one of the parents and that the characteristics of the other parent were not discernable in the hybrid. The traits were stable from one generation to the next. He further discovered that the seven traits were inherited as separate "units", (Mendelian factors) that would later be called genes. Mendel had studied mathematics and physics at the university in Vienna, and by using statistical calculations, he was able to characterise the pattern of inheritance, making him one of the first to apply statistical methods to biology. By using mathematical and statistical calculations, he was able to establish that each of the parents had one pair of factors for every trait and that the hybrid inherited one of these factors from each parent. He introduced the concept of dominant and recessive patterns of heredity.

Mendel's publication from 1865, *Versuche über Plantzen-Hybriden* (*Experiments on Plant Hybridization*), is considered to be one of the three most important publications in biology together with Darwin's *On the*

The Hunt for the Parathyroids, First Edition. Jörgen Nordenström.
© 2013 John Wiley & Sons, Ltd. Published 2013 by John Wiley & Sons, Ltd.

Origin of Species by Means of Natural Selection (1859) and Watson's and Crick's article on the DNA double-helix from 1953. Mendel's findings were, however, difficult for other people to understand. He sent his report to more than 100 institutions and researchers throughout Europe, but his discovery was given very little attention. Mendel was simply ahead of his time and his contemporaries were not ready to accept his observations.

The monks at the monastery in Brno burnt Mendel's notebooks, manuscripts and scientific books shortly after his death in 1884. His discovery was largely overlooked and it was not until 35 years after Mendel had published his work that three European researchers took notice of his findings. Mendel was vindicated, and today is regarded as one of the great scientists in biology and the father of genetics. DNA was identified as early as 1871, but it took many years before genetic research dealing with human biology gained some impetus. In 1944 Oswald Avery showed that the Mendelian factors, the genes, were made up of DNA, and several years later when Watson and Crick presented their model of the genetic code with nucleic acids shaped in a double helix, the doors opened for molecular biology. There was certainly substance to Crick's proud statement "We have discovered the secret of life."

When the Human Genome Project managed to identify and establish the order of the genes in the human genome, Francis Collins, the head of the project, described this as having discovered the Language of God. The unique language of biology had been deciphered in the same way that archaeologists had earlier succeeded in understanding Egyptian hieroglyphics. The Genome Project demonstrated that the human genome was made up of 30 000 different genes and 3 billion base pairs, but that only 500 000 DNA segments showed variations between different individuals that could be of potential interest for identifying a risk of disease. Human DNA was shown to be 98.4% identical to that of the chimpanzee. Charting the human genome paved the way for studies on the links between the changes in the genome and the risks of developing diseases, such as for different kinds of cancer, cardiovascular and neurological diseases. In a longer perspective there is a potential for creating a greater understanding of various disease mechanisms and to develop new medicines.

Great strides were made during the 1970s and 1980s in charting the function of the parathyroids, the molecular and biological mechanisms that steer the regulation of calcium and the understanding of parathyroid disorders. The regulatory system for the metabolism of calcium was shown to be so sophisticated that a change of only a few percent in the calcium ion levels causes a change many times over in parathyroid hormone secretion: increasing when the calcium levels are lowered and decreasing when the calcium concentration increases. Minute changes of 1–2% in the parathyroid hormone levels are enough to initiate effects in this extremely sensitive system. The supply of parathyroid hormone in the parathyroid glands is sufficient to respond to an increased hormone demand for 1–2 hours, but if the calcium level is very low new production of parathyroid hormone can begin after just 20–30 minutes. If calcium deficiency persists for a long period of time, dormant cells are recruited and transformed into active hormone producers. Increased parathyroid hormone production may also develop as result of a chronic stimulation. The end result is an increased production of parathyroid hormone due to an increase in the amount of parathyroid tissue. This can be caused by chronic kidney disease, where the amount of parathyroid tissue can be 5–10 times greater than normal. Other mechanisms for maintaining normal calcium levels are found in the kidneys where calcium is filtered through the system of small tubules, and the majority is reabsorbed into the bloodstream. If there is a surplus or a deficiency of calcium, the kidneys can regulate the levels by varying the secretion of calcium in the urine.

The skeleton contains 99% of all the calcium in the body. Parathyroid hormone and vitamin D can regulate the mobilisation of calcium from the skeleton into the bloodstream. This mobilisation can be so pronounced with elevated parathyroid hormone levels (in hyperparathyroidism) that osteoporosis and a deterioration of bone quality occurs. In hyperparathyroidism there is a change in the relationship between parathyroid hormone and calcium concentrations preventing the hormone levels being reduced. A kind of hormone resistance or a hormone insensitivity occurs that demands abnormally high calcium levels to lower the production of parathyroid hormone (in other words there is a higher set point for parathyroid hormone).

There were data as early as 1960 indicating that calcium had a direct effect on the parathyroid cell, and that it could regulate the production and secretion of the hormone by means of an unknown process. However, it would take another 20 years before it was possible to chart this thermostat-like mechanism – the calcium-sensing receptor (CaSR) – that relays signals about the calcium levels in the environment surrounding the cells to the cells' internal milieu. This "calciostat" is wedged into the cell like a cork in a bottle and it consists of three parts: one part is outside of the cell, one is in the cell wall and one part reaches into the inside of the cell. Calcium-sensing receptors are found on the surfaces of the cells in the parathyroids, the kidneys, and in the skeleton. When calcium binds to the receptor on the surface of the parathyroid cell, calcium ions are released inside the cell. The calcium-sensing receptors regulate the function of the parathyroid cell by affecting the secretion and production of parathyroid hormone and the production of new active parathyroid cells. The calcium-sensing receptors belong to the category of G protein-coupled receptors (GPCRs). GPCRs are a super-family of proteins that can be found in nearly all of the organs of the body, and they work like signal systems for many substances, including amino acids, proteins, fats, hormones and ions. The receptors also react to tastes and smells, and even to light and drugs. When a matching substance, a ligand, is bound to a receptor on the surface of the cell, the receptor protein changes its form and a signal is generated inside the cell. This signal starts a pre-programmed cellular process. In this way the environment outside of the cell can communicate with the inner milieu of the cell.

After the chemical structure of the parathyroid hormone became known, it still remained to be shown how the signal system worked on a cellular level. It was shown that the hormone worked via a GPCR receptor, known as the PTH1 receptor, in a similar way to calcium's cellular receptor. The PTH1 receptor exists mainly in bone and kidney cells and the hormone regulates the calcium levels of the blood by mobilising or absorbing calcium in the skeleton, and by increasing or decreasing the secretion of calcium via the kidneys. In addition to the PTH1 receptor, there is also a PTH2 receptor (expressed in brain tissue). Recently a PTH3 receptor has been identified activated by fragments of the hormone's "tail" (the C-terminal end of the hormone's amino acid chain). The PTH3 receptors have the opposite effect of the classic PTH1 receptors, that is, the activation of the tail receptor lowers the calcium levels of the blood instead of raising them.

GPCRs comprise at least three different classes or families which have a large number of physiological effects relevant for a variety of diseases. The calcium-sensing receptor belongs to the so-called B-family and the PTH receptors belong to the C-family. The pharmaceutical industry is extremely interested in these receptors, and it has been estimated that about half of all new drugs work via their effects on different GPCR families. Nearly 400 pharmaceutically interesting GPCRs have been identified, but many of them are described as "orphans" because their exact importance has not yet been established. They are still waiting for a family into which they can be placed, and maybe even a disease to treat. If you were to make a wild guess about the mechanism steering the effect of a new drug, you would have the best chance of arriving at the right answer if you guessed GPCR. The pharmaceutical industry is enthusiastic – "*It's a GPCR World*." Drugs that work via GPCRs include *Claritin* (an antihistamine for treating pollen allergies), *Zantac* (an acid inhibitor for stomach ulcers) and *Zyprexa* (a mood stabiliser for schizophrenia).

Even before the structure of the calcium-sensing receptors was known, substances that could increase the calcium concentration inside of the parathyroid cell had been identified. Known as calcimimetics, they were

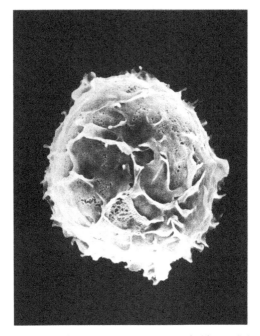

Figure 11.1 Parathyroid cell, magnification x7500. (Used with permission from Lennart Nilsson)

shown to work by activating the calcium-sensing receptors. By creating calcium-like effects, they increase the sensitivity to calcium of the receptor. *Cinacalcet* is a drug that has been on the market for some years and can be used to treat patients with renal failure who have developed compensatory enlarged parathyroid glands with increased parathyroid hormone production. *Cinacalcet* can also be used in patients with classical hyperparathyroidism not fit for surgery.

Parathyroid hormone and its function have thus been shown to be more sophisticated than anyone could have imagined from the start. The complexity can be seen as a reflection of the very important role that calcium plays in most of the body's cells and cell functions. The complex interaction of calcium, parathyroid hormone, and the target organs ultimately provide high tolerance of minor deviations from normal values. The system is very accurate as major, life-threatening metabolic errors are very rare in actual fact.

It makes one wonder about the complexity of the human body and how well such a complicated system can work for most people. Day after day and year after year there are thousands of different systems operating and interacting with one another so that normal functions can be maintained in spite of variations in the external environment. There are many older people today with no serious diseases or severe ailments, and it is amazing that humans, sometimes for even 100 years or more, can have life functions that remain so relatively problem-free.

The traditional view of ageing is that many functions work less effectively as time goes on. Examples of this are decreasing muscle strength, worn-out joints, and the cessation of menstruation with menopause when there are no more eggs to recruit, and deteriorating eyesight. Almost like an old car that rusts away and gradually runs down until it just stops running. Yet there is another process in ageing that keeps very important functions in the body from drastically changing over time. Instead they continue working fully until they stop completely, after which they are replaced by a reserve mechanism – a backup system. When this stops working in turn, the next reserve mechanism takes over, and so on. This does not mean that all of the complex systems have worked perfectly all of the time in very old people, but many systems can stop working and be replaced by a reserve mechanism. These backup systems ensure that important processes can be retained. This reserve equipment might not function as well as the original parts, and it may not provide as much preparedness for major disruptions or strains, but it tends to work well on the whole. When all of the reserve mechanisms have been used, one reaches the end of the road. This entire process is steered to some extent by different genes and also by self-regulatory mechanisms.

There are hereditary changes in the calcium-sensing receptors that either lead to elevated or lowered calcium levels in the blood. Familial hypocalciuric hypercalcaemia (FHH) is a rare hereditary calcium disorder that can be difficult to differentiate from hyperparathyroidism. In this condition, the individual is asymptomatic and does not require surgery, but has low calcium levels in the urine and high concentrations of calcium in the blood. The cause is a mutation on chromosome 3. The calcium-sensing receptor is partially inactivated in this condition – the calciostat is raised – which means that higher than normal calcium levels are needed to inhibit the parathyroids' hormone producing cells. Since the elevated levels of calcium in the blood are due to a receptor defect, the elevated calcium levels cannot be normalised by performing a parathyroid operation. The concepts of FHH, and even the underlying causes of the elevated calcium levels in the blood, were unknown until the beginning of the 1980s. Prior to that time there were people with FHH who had undergone a number of parathyroid operations because elevated calcium values had been detected. Elevated calcium values that persisted in spite of repeated operations were considered to be a challenge ever since the first operations in the 1920s and many surgeons thought it to be the test of a master to normalise the calcium levels in these patients that were assumed to have hyperparathyroidism. There were individuals who had many operations (sometimes as many as half a dozen) in the search for a cure for a condition that today cannot even be characterised as a disease. In most of these earlier cases of FHH the surgeons managed to finally remove all parathyroid tissue, whereupon the calcium fell to levels that were much too low. These individuals thereby acquired a chronic parathyroid hormone deficiency and became dependent upon lifelong treatment with vitamin D in order to maintain sufficient calcium levels. A careful survey of the family history and a genetic analysis can identify these patients with elevated blood calcium levels so that an unnecessary operation can be avoided. A middle-aged woman with elevated calcium levels related the following story:

> "My brother was operated on several years ago for hyperparathy-roidism, and even though three and a half parathyroid glands were removed, his calcium values the day after the operation were just as high as they had been before the operation."

This single sentence is an illuminating description of a family with FHH. There are probably several hundred families in the world in which FHH occurs.

The human parathyroid hormone gene is located on chromosome 11 and is regulated by several different substances including calcium, phosphate and vitamin D. Although many changes in the human genome do not cause changes in function, there are characteristic gene changes that affect the regulation of calcium as well as the growth of the parathyroids and the function of parathyroid hormone. In 80–85% of all cases of hyperparathyroidism, there is a benign enlargement of a single gland (an adenoma). In the remaining cases there are several enlarged glands (multiple adenomas) or a diffuse enlargement of them all (hyperplasia). The existence of a parathyroid cancer is extremely rare. Chronic kidney disease, lithium treatment, or previous radiation treatment of the neck region can all cause hyperparathyroidism, but apart from these there are no other known external factors that can lead to the disease. Hyperparathyroidism can have a hereditary background in patients, often relatively young ones. In these hereditary disorders there are changes in the genome, and so far four genes have been identified that can lead to hyperparathyroidism: MEN1 (chromosome 11); HRPT2 (chromosome 1); CASR (chromosome 3); and RET (chromosome 10).

For a long time it was unclear why patients with a hereditary disposition to hyperparathyroidism would develop the disease over time. In 1971 the cancer researcher Alfred Knudson presented the hypothesis that cancer can occur as a result of repeated mutations in the DNA of a cell. According to this model, a cancerous growth can develop when both of the genes in a chromosome pair have undergone mutations. People who inherit a mutated gene from one of their parents (a first hit) have to be affected by another mutation (a second hit) in the other chromosome pair in order for tumour development to begin. This hypothesis, the "two-hit" theory of cancer development, is based upon the occurrence of repeated mutations – lightning has to strike the same house twice. The hypothesis has been shown to hold true for both cancer tumours and benign enlargements such as in the parathyroid glands. Knudson's hypothesis can also explain the start of hyperparathyroidism since an increased volume of the parathyroid glands causes an increase in the production of parathyroid hormone. It was later shown that the development of certain tumours could be caused by an activation of oncogenes (genes that stimulate cell growth) as well as by a silencing of tumour-suppressing genes. A first hit in an oncogene does not necessarily lead to the development of cancer or a gland enlargement as long as the corresponding tumour suppressor gene is intact. Conversely, a mutated tumour suppressor gene does not have to lead to cancer as long as the oncogene has not been activated.

Vitamin D, different vitamin D receptor genes and the gene for the calcium-sensing receptor (CaSR) all play key roles in the regulation of calcium and parathyroid hormone. Low blood calcium, low vitamin D levels and a high blood phosphate concentration, as well as a decreased expression of the vitamin D receptor or CaSR can all cause the parathyroid cells to grow. These changes increase the risk of a genetic mutation (a "hit") which can lead to hyperparathyroidism.

Knudson's "two-hit theory" can also be applied to benign parathyroid enlargements with a hereditary component. Radiation in the neck region can be a mutation risk, a possible "hit." Mutations probably seldom occur, and repeated mutations are even rarer. Individuals that have already in-herited a mutation, a first "hit," have a greater risk of developing hyper-parathyroidism if another mutation happens to occur. This explains why heredity-related hyperparathyroidism occurs in relatively young persons, and why they are at greater risk of having tumours in more than one parathyroid gland.

Today there are a number of known heredity-related varieties of hyper-parathyroidism, all of which are rare: MEN1 and MEN2A (multiple endocrine neoplasia); FIHPT (familial isolated hyperparathyroidism); FHH (familial hypocalciuric hypercalcaemia); ADMH (autosomal dominant mild hyperparathyroidism) and HPT-JT (hyperparathyroid jaw tumour).

Several of the hereditary forms of hyperparathyroidism were described long before the concept was established or the mechanisms behind the inheritance became known. In 1884 Davies-Colley described a hyperparathyroid jaw tumour in a 13-year-old girl who had died of a "strange skeletal disease." Among other things, the girl had a tumour on her jaw, a compressed spine that caused paralysis in both her arms and legs, and kidney stones. It is remarkable that Davies-Colley did chemical analyses and could establish that the amount of calcium in the urine was high – an observation that preceded the studies that Fuller Albright and others did more than 40 years later on patients with hyperparathyroidism. Another early observation of hereditary hyperparathyroidism with MEN1 was made by Jacob Erdheim in 1903.

Chapter 12 **The pharmacological paradox**

A calcium-deficient skeleton and fractures were the first observable signs of disease in the parathyroid glands, the classic picture that appeared when too much parathyroid hormone circulated in the blood. The hormone was therefore considered to be a destructive (catabolic) hormone that did more damage than good when it was present in excess. Considering this, it seems paradoxical that parathyroid hormone has been shown to be effective in the treatment of osteoporosis.

During evolution, single cells and simple organisms developed into more complex and larger structures. Calcium became indispensible for supporting cell wall stability and cytoskeletal architecture of all cells, to form bone to provide mechanical support for load-bearing and locomotion, for teeth to facilitate food intake and for attack/defence purposes, and for the protection of vulnerable internal structures. The calcium ion has a number of chemical characteristics that are favourable for structural elements, namely its large size, its ability to coordinate in a variety of geometries and to display high coordination numbers, putting it at an advantage in acting as a cross-linking agent in biology. Cross-links mediated by calcium ions are reversible and therefore responsive to changes of conditions; an important characteristic, for example, for load-bearing structures. Early in history, humans made use of calcium's properties related to structure, such as the use of mortar, cements and concretes as building materials derived from calcium-rich rocks (marble and limestone). Animals and plants have also made widespread use of calcium carbonate, the main component of shells in the marine world, snails, pearls, corals and eggs. In vertebrates, calcium phosphate (hydroxyapatite) is the main component of bones and teeth.

For a long time bone was considered to be a passive tissue responding mainly to hormonal and dietary influences but research during the last

---

The Hunt for the Parathyroids, First Edition. Jörgen Nordenström.
© 2013 John Wiley & Sons, Ltd. Published 2013 by John Wiley & Sons, Ltd.

century has shown bone to be a highly dynamic tissue responding to metabolic and mechanical demands as well as a reservoir of storage for calcium and phosphate. Thus, bone is not just a static structural support for our body but a flexible living tissue and an important tool for the maintenance of stable calcium concentrations in the blood stream.

Osteoporosis is characterised by reduced bone density and altered bone composition. These changes weaken the skeleton and increase the risk of fractures. Osteoporosis is a widespread disease in the Western world, and it has been estimated that close to 4 million osteoporosis-related fractures occur annually in Europe, costing 30 billion Euros. The most common locations of osteoporotic fractures are the wrists, hips and spine. Hip fractures carry the greatest disease burden of the osteoporosis-related fractures, where 50% of the patients who suffer hip fractures are unable to walk without support, 25% are dependent upon assistance and 20% will die from fracture-associated complications within one year. The annual number of global deaths caused by hip fractures is estimated to be 750 000. Osteoporotic fractures are thus associated with an enormous burden of disability for the patients and their families, making them a massive problem for society.

In osteoporosis, the skeleton's diminished ability to withstand stress and external force is the result of an altered bone metabolism, there is a higher rate of breakdown of bone tissue than the rate of formation of new bone. This leads to decreased bone density and a decrease in total bone mass. Bone tissue normally undergoes a continuous renewal process through the breakdown of existing bone tissue with the aid of special bone resorbing cells (osteoclasts) along with the formation of new bone by another specialised type of bone cells (osteoblasts). In osteoporosis there is a negative balance between bone resorption and the formation of new bone, and there is often an increase in the rate of bone transformation.

In the mid-19th century when population studies first discovered that osteoporosis was a common disorder, the methods of treatment were limited and mainly consisted of recommendations for a well-balanced diet, regular exercise, calcium and vitamin D supplements, and oestrogen for postmenopausal women. A second generation of drugs was later developed, the bisphosphonates, whose main effect was to reduce the activity of the osteoclasts (the cells that caused the breakdown of bone). This resulted in a change in the negative balance between the breakdown and the formation of the skeleton. These anti-resorptive drugs were only moderately effective and usually resulted in a 2–4% increase in bone density. This treatment had a limited effect and few patients were able to regain a normal bone mineral density. The pharmaceutical industry continued to try to develop substances with different mechanisms of action and greater effects.

As early as 1929, Bauer, Albright and Aub observed that giving parathyroid hormone to laboratory animals over an extended period of time led to a gradual reduction of the hormone's ability to mobilise calcium from the skeleton. It was assumed that some kind of immunity or resistance to the hormone developed after longer treatments. This was thought to be "unfortunate" considering the potential uses of the hormone as a medicine for treating parathyroid hormone deficiencies and even lead poisoning. It was also noted that the long-term treatment of laboratory animals with parathyroid hormone increased the animals' bone mass, an observation that was laconically commented upon by saying, "this could not be explained."

A few years later, Hans Selye began studying the previously observed phenomenon of immunity or resistance to parathyroid hormone observed by Aub's research team. Selye was of Austro-Hungarian descent and had received a Rockefeller grant for research studies in North America. He began his studies at Johns Hopkins, but he had difficulty adapting to the informal climate there. Instead, he joined James Collip's research team at McGill University in Montreal where he felt the environment was more "European," that is, more comparable to his own background. Collip was running many research projects and he assigned Selye to the task of studying the effects of parathyroid hormone on bone tissue. Selye discovered with his studies on rats that the reason the calcium-mobilising effect of the hormone diminished over time had nothing to do with the development of resistance. Instead, the explanation was that long-term parathyroid hormone treatment led to increased activity of the osteoblasts (which increase the formation of new bone), but not to an increase in the number of osteoclasts (which break down bone), as many had assumed earlier. This resulted in the formation of new bone tissue. Since the elevated parathyroid hormone levels in hyper-parathyroidism caused an increase in the breakdown of bone, it was assumed that Selye's observations in rats had no relevance to human medicine. It would take more than 40 years before this observation would be brought to light as the basis for parathyroid hormone's role as a potential drug for treating osteoporosis.

Collip's, and also Selye's, interest in parathyroid hormone waned. Instead they began research on a possible hormonal interrelationship between the pituitary gland and the ovaries. Collip tried to identify a new ovarian hormone and Selye was given the task of collecting ovaries in Montreal's slaughterhouse to be used for the isolation of the prospective hormone. They failed to find a new ovarian hormone and Selye noted with disappointment that many of the animals that had been injected with the ovarian extract became ill and some even died. When they were dissected, they had enlarged adrenal glands and stomach ulcers. Frustrated by this discovery, Selye injected some animals with formaldehyde (a solution used to preserve biological specimens) and discovered that similar organ changes appeared. In experiments that today would be considered unthinkable, he exposed rats to extreme heat and cold, bright blinking lights after the rats' eyelids had been sewn open, or extreme physical exertion where the animals had to swim in water tanks until they nearly collapsed. After these extreme experiments he found that the animals showed the same organ changes that had been observed after injections of ovarian extract or formaldehyde. He called these organ responses due to extreme external influences an "alarm reaction," and he later identified several stages in the pattern of reactions (alarm, resistance, exhaustion). Selye studied the mechanisms behind these phenomena which he called the "general adaptation syndrome" and he found that the effects were caused by an increase in the activity of the pituitary gland that stimulated the adrenal gland to secrete steroid hormones that had an anti-inflammatory effect. If the animal's pituitary gland had been removed before the experiments, the characteristic organ changes did not occur. However if the adrenal gland had been removed the normal reaction patterns could be restored by giving the animal adrenal extract. Both an intact pituitary function and an intact adrenal function were apparently necessary for this reaction pattern to occur.

One of Selye's studies demonstrated that administering adrenal extract to laboratory animals increased their resistance to oxygen depletion. In 1941, the American intelligence service discovered that Germany had purchased large quantities of beef adrenal glands from Argentina. This started a rumor that the Luftwaffe's pilots by taking adrenal extracts, could fly at an altitude of 40 000 feet, an altitude that would make it impossible to stop a German air raid. This rumour was enough to make the American government allocate large sums of money to research groups that were busy developing and purifying "*Substance E*," which would later be given the name *cortisone*.

Ever since the days of Hippocrates, medical students have been taught that every disease has a specific cause and a specific course. This was the actual foundation of the art of medicine: specific diseases required specific treatments. What Selye had shown was something entirely different, namely that different types of extreme external stress could induce identical organ changes. Selye used the word "stress" to describe the phenomenon. He would later come to partly regret that he had chosen the term "stress", and he admitted that he probably would have used another term for the phenomenon if his knowledge of English had been better. In physics the word stress has a specific meaning that pertains to the ability of a substance to return to its original state after being subjected to external forces. Selye's concept of stress generated a lot of attention early on and it came to be used colloquially to describe not only the physical or mental strain, but also the actual reactions to such challenges and the final effect as well. When the Nobel Prize was to be awarded in 1955, Selye remained a candidate up until the final round. However, the person who was finally awarded the prize for his enzyme research was a Swede, Hugo Theorell.

Now let's get back to the hormone of this small organ. The explanation for how chronic elevated levels of parathyroid hormone could cause the mobilisation of calcium from the skeleton while daily injections of the hormone could stimulate the formation of new bone would not be understood until long into the 1970s. The appearance of the highly sensitive RIA method for determining parathyroid hormone levels made it possible to study the hormone's normal diurnal variations in the body. Studies were made in which the parathyroid hormone concentration in the blood of healthy individuals was measured at regular intervals over a 24-hour period. This revealed that the levels showed a periodicity. During the daytime parathyroid hormone levels were stable, but they began to rise early in the evening and reached their highest level late at night and then decreased to the base level in the morning. They increased by 50–100% at night. In hyperparathyroidism the normal daily rhythm is attenuated, and there is a high and constant secretion of parathyroid hormone which potentiates the hormone's effect of bone mobilisation. The result of this can be, after many years, osteoporosis or in extreme cases, *osteitis fibrosa cystica* – the most pronounced skeletal manifestation of hyperparathyroidism.

The periodic fluctuations in biological systems that occur over a 24-hour period are called circadian rhythms, from the Latin *circa* (around) and *dies* (day). A circadian rhythm is a physiological process that returns to its starting point after a certain amount of time. Daily rhythms and profiles of basal and stimulated secretions of several hormones are common in all biological systems. They are usually adjusted to a 24-hour period and operate rhythmically under stable conditions such as the intake of food and light/darkness. Human daily rhythms include temperature, enzymatic and hormonal rhythms. The centre of the biological clock is located in two suprachiasmatic nuclei found in the hypothalamus. This centre of the biological clock is stimulated by external light that hits the retina of the eye. The clock is not exactly adjusted to 24 hours but is closer to 25 hours. The external influences of different factors, *zeitgebers*, finely tune the clock to 24 hours. The most important factors in this process are the daily cycle of light and darkness and the routines for sleeping and being awake. The biological clock can be adjusted by about two hours per day, allowing most biological processes to readily adapt to slight changes in the daily routine. After quickly moving across several time zones in a transatlantic flight, for instance, it takes several days for the biological clock to re-adjust and get back into sync, something we experience as jet lag. In addition to the central part of the biological clock, there are a large number of clock genes that regulate the different biological processes in the body. The body's biological clock and the circadian rhythms play an important role in most bodily functions and, in terms of developmental biology, they are seen as a way of saving resources so that all of the different systems do not have to be running during every hour of the day. Certain manifestations of diseases that occur at particular times of day (asthma and sudden cardiac arrest in the morning, sickle cell crises in the afternoon, epilepsy in the evening) can be explained by effects initiated by the biological clock. The clock makes it possible to calculate or 'measure' time. Migrating birds use their biological clocks, together with the positions of the sun and the stars, to navigate the flight patterns to their nesting places or winter habitats.

Aub and Selye's observations regarding parathyroid hormone's anabolic effects of building up bone tissue were followed by animal tests during the 1970s. For a long time it was hard to understand how a daily injection of parathyroid hormone could be anabolic for bone and increase bone density. The explanation for the phenomenon was shown to be that a brief increase of the parathyroid hormone levels in the blood for a period of up to two hours stimulated primitive bone cells to develop into osteoblasts without causing a parallel activation of the destructive cells, the osteoclasts. It was found that the osteoblasts, but not osteoclasts, were found to have parathyroid hormone receptors that react to elevated parathyroid hormone levels. A brief stimulation of high circulating parathyroid hormone does not activate local growth factors and cell factors (cytokines) in the osteoblasts, so no new osteoclasts are recruited and no bone resorption is initiated. Parathyroid hormone also increases the life span of the osteoblasts by decreasing programmed cell-death (apoptosis). Osteoclasts are activated only by a longer period of parathyroid hormone stimulation. This entire complex activating process of osteoclast activity (the RANK-L/RANK/osteoprotegerin pathway) is not initiated when there is only a brief parathyroid hormone stimulation. So "timing is everything" when it comes to bone metabolism. Continuous elevation of parathyroid hormone in the blood stream leads to bone loss while intermittent short elevations of the hormone can be anabolic for bone.

These fundamental discoveries led to clinical studies in which the possibilities of parathyroid hormone treatment for osteoporosis were examined and the effects proved to be remarkable. In a study from the beginning of the present century, R.M. Neer and his colleagues examined 1600 patients with vertebral osteoporosis. In this study daily injections of parathyroid hormone increased bone mass in the lower back by 13%, and reduced the risk of vertebral compression by almost 70%. Increased bone mass and reduced fracture risk was also seen in other parts of the skeleton. Two different variants of parathyroid hormone exist today as registered drugs for the treatment of osteoporosis: *Forsteo (teriparatide)* consisting of fragments 1–34 of the hormone and *Preotact* which consists of the full-length hormone (1–84). It has also recently been shown that daily injections of PTH can speed up the healing process by 19% in patients with wrist fractures.

Parathyroid hormone has thus proven itself to be a remarkable hormone. Its normal function is necessary in order to maintain normal function in almost every cell in the body. A total lack of the hormone leads to death, chronic hyperfunction causes disease and, in the worst cases, premature death; and yet paradoxically the hormone can also be used as a drug to treat osteoporosis and improve healing of fractures.

Is this the end of the medical expedition studying the tiny organ that Sandström discovered and its hormone? Sixty years ago Fuller Albright wrote in his monograph, *The Parathyroid Glands and Metabolic Bone Disease*:

> "In the final analysis very little is known about anything, and much that seems true today turns out to be only partly true tomorrow."

This quotation is probably just as valid today as it was when it was written.

> "For the Snark's a peculiar creature, that won't
> Be caught in a commonplace way.
> Do all that you know, and try all that you don't:
> Not a chance must be wasted to-day!"
>
> Lewis Carroll, *The Hunting of the Snark*,
> Fit the Fourth

The adventure continues.

References and notes

General references

Albright F, Ellsworth R. *Uncharted Seas*. Portland: Kalmia Press, 1990.

Bilezikian JP, Marcus R, Levine MA (eds.) *The Parathyroids. Basic and Clinical Concepts*. 2nd ed. San Diego: Academic Press, 2001.

Boothby WM. The parathyroid glands: a review of the literature. *Endocrinology* 1921; 5:403–40.

Bryson B. *A Short History of Nearly Everything*. London: Black Swan, 2004.

Carney JA. The glandulae parathyroidea of Ivar Sandström. Contributions from two continents. *Am J Surg Path* 1996; 20:1123–44.

Clark OH, Duh Q-Y, Kebebew E (eds.) *Textbook of Endocrine Surgery*. 2nd ed. Philadelphia: Elsevier Saunders, 2005.

Le Fanu J. *The Rise and Fall of Modern Medicine*. London: Abacus, 2000.

Ochsner AJ, Thomson RL. *The Surgery and Pathology of the Thyroid and Parathyroid Glands*. London: Georger Keener & Co, 1910.

Potts JT. Parathyroid hormone: past and present. *J Endocrinol* 2005; 187:311–25.

Thomson N. The history of hyperparathyroidism. *Acta Chir Scand* 1990; 156:5–21.

Welbourn RB. *The History of Endocrine Surgery*. New York: Praeger, 1990.

Introduction

p.x.   Bernard C. *An Introduction to the Study of Experimental Medicine*. New York: Dover Publ., 1957.

xi.   Carroll L. *The Hunting of the Snark*. London: Macmillan, 1876.

1. Sandström's discovery

p.1.   Sandström I. Om en ny körtel hos meniskan och åtskilliga däggdjur. *Upsala Läkareförenings Förhandlingar*. 1880; band XV (nr 7 & 8):441–71.

The Hunt for the Parathyroids, First Edition. Jörgen Nordenström.
© 2013 John Wiley & Sons, Ltd. Published 2013 by John Wiley & Sons, Ltd.

Sandström's article is available in English: Seipel CM. *On a New Gland in Man and Several Animals.* Baltimore: The Johns Hopkins Press, 1938.

5. Remak R. *Untersuchungen über die Entvicklung der Wirbelthiere.* Berlin: G Reimer, 1855, p.191.

Virchow R. *Die Krankhaften Geschülste.* Berlin: A. Hirchwald, 1863. Band iii, p.13. DA Welch (Concerning the parathyroid glands: a critical,anatomical and experimental study. *J Anat Physiol* 1898; 32: 292–307) states that the following investigators have observed the parathyroids prior to Sandström: Gruber, Verneuil, Callender, Bruch, Porta, Simon, Paget, Kroenlein, Poland, Kadyi, Zuckerkandl, Madelung, Wölfer, Wagner, Fuhr, Carle, Wolf, Semon, Piana, Ewald, Autokratow, Gibson, and others.

6. Bryson B. *A Short History of Nearly Everything.* London: Black Swan, 2004, p. 453–5.

7. Hammar JA. Glandula parathyreoidea (Sandström). *Hygea. Festband* 1908; 42:1–24.

Shattock SG. The parathyroids in Graves's disease. *BMJ* 1905; 30 Dec:1694–95.

8. Owen R. On the anatomy of the Indian Rhinoceros (Rh. Unicornis, L.). *Trans Zool Soc Lond* 1862; 4:31–58.

Ridley G. *Clara's Grand Tour.* New York: Atlantic Monthly Press, 2004.

Rookmaaker LC. *The Rhinoceros in Captivity. A List of 2439 Rhinoceros Kept From Roman Times to 1994.* Haag: SPB Academic Publishing, 1998, p. 85–6.

Felger EA, Zeiger MA. The death of an Indian rhinoceros. *World J Surg* 2010; 34:1805–10.

Carney JA. The glandulae parathyroidea of Ivar Sandström. Contributions from two continents. *Am J Surg Path* 1996; 20:1123–44.

10. Nuland S.The fundamental units of life: Sick cells, microscopes and Rudolph Virchow. In: *Doctors.* New York: Vintage Books, 1998.

11. Robb-Smith AHT. Papa Virchow. *Lancet* 1958; 272:851.

Meyers MA. *Happy Accidents. Serendipity in Modern Medical Breakthroughs.* New York: Arcade Publ. 2007, p.306.

Yalow R. Radioimmunoassay: A probe for the fine structure of biological systems. *The Nobel Prizes 1977.* Stockholm: Almqvist & Wiksell International. 1978, p. 236–64.

Sandström's publication was noted as abstracts in three German medical yearbooks:

Retzius G. *Hofmann-Schwalbe's Jahresberichte ü d Fortschr. Anat u Physiol.*1880. Band IX: 224–6.

Berger W. Ueber eine neue Drüse beim Menschen und bei verschiedenen Säugethieren. *Schmidt's Jahrbücher des In- und Ausländischen gesammten Medicin.* Leipzig, 1880. Band 187, Ref. No. 384:114–18.

Kollmann J. *Virchow-Hirsch's Jahresbericht über Die Leistungen und Fortschritte in Der Gesammten Medicin. Erste Abreilung: Anathomie und Physiologie.* Berlin, 1881.Band 1, XV Jahrgang: 11–12.

12. Toobin J. Google's Moon Shot. *The New Yorker*, 5 February, 2007.

Vise DA. *The Google Story*. London: Pan Books, 2006.

Kelly K. Scan this book. *The New York Times*, 14 May, 2006.

13. Ask-Upmark E, Rexed B, Sandström B. Ivar Sandström and the parathyroid glands. *Acta Universit. Upsaliensis* 1967; 7–13.

16. *Söderhamns Tidning*, 3 June, 1889.

2. Unexpected problems

p.18. Recklinghausen F. *Die Fibröse oder deformierende Osteitis, osteomalacie und osteoplastische Carcinose*. Featschrift für R v. Virchow, Berlin, 1891.

19. Cook M, Molto E, Anderson C. Possible case of hyperparathyroidism in a Roman period skeleton from Dakhleh oasis, Egypt, diagnosed using bone histomorphometry. *Am J Physic Anthropol* 1988; 75:23–30.

di Santi P. Parathyroidgeschwulst Symptome von Maligner Erkrankung des Larynx hervorrufend. Operation und Heilung. *Internat Centralbl f Laryngol, Rhinol u Verwandte Wissenschaften* 1900; 16:546–7.

Benjamins CE. Ueber die Glandulae parathyreoidea (Epitelkörperchen). *Ziegler's Beitrage* 1902; Band 31:143–82.

Askanasy M. Ueber Osteitis deformans ohne osteoides Gewebe. *Arbeiten aus dem Gebeite der pathologischen Anat u Bakteriol dem pathol-Anatom. Inst zu Tübingen*, 1904; Band 4, heft 3:398–422.

Goris C. Exstirpation de trois lobules parathyroïdiens kystigues. *Annales de la Société Belge de Chirurgie*, 1905; 8:394–95.

Delbridge LW, Palazzo FF. First parathyroid surgeon: Sir John Bland-Sutton and the parathyroids. *ANZ J Surg* 2007; 77:1058–61.

Bland-Sutton J. *Tumours Innocent and Malignant*. 6th ed. New York: Paul B. Hoebber, 1917.

20. Warren S. *Passages from the Diary of a Late Physician*. Reprinted in: Blackwood's Magazine, 1830. Amsterdam: Fredonia Books, 2005.

21. Rutledge RH. In commemoration of Theodor Billroth on the 150th anniversary of his birth. *Surgery* 1979; 86:672–93.

24. Mayo CH. Goitre: with preliminary report of one hundred and eighty-two operations upon the thyroid. *Trans South Surg Gynecol Assoc* 1905; 18:145–66.

25. Wölfler A. Wietere Beiträge zur chirurgischen Behandlung des Kropfes. *Wien Med Wochenschr* 1879; 28:758–60.

27. Kirklin JW. The middle 1950s and Walter Lillehai. *J Thorac Cardiovasc Surg* 1989; 98:822–4.

Erdheim J. Über die Dentinverkalkung im Nagezahn bei der Epithelkörperchentransplantation. *Frankfurter Zeitschr f Pathol* 1911; vii:295–347.

28. Eiselsberg A. Ueber erfogreiche Einheilung der Katzschilddruse in die Bauchdecke und Auftreten von Tetanie nach deren Exstirpation. *Wien Klin Wochenschr* 1892; 5:81–85.

Eiselsberg A. Ueber Wachsthums-Störungen bei Tieren nach frühzeitiger Schilddrüsen-Exstirpation. *Arch f Klin Chir* 1895; Bd. XLIX, Heft 1:1–31.

3. The age of glorious discoveries

p.32. Fröman N. *Marie and Pierre Curie and the discovery of Polonium and Radium*. www.nobelprize.org

33. Curie È. *Madame Curie: A Biography*. New York: Da Capo Press, 1937.
35. Personal communication, S. James Adelstein.

4. A gland in search of a function

p.37. Krause W. *Nachträge zur allgemeinen und mikroskopishe Anatomie*. Hahn, Hannover, 1881.

Krause W. *Die Anatomie des Kaninschens*. Leipzig: Verlag von Wilhelm Engelmann. 2nd ed., 1884.

38. Gley E. Sur les fonctions de la thyroide chez le lapin et chez le chien. *Compt Rend de Soc de Biol* 1891; seance 12 December; 3:843–7.

Gley E. Sur les fonctions du corps thyroide. *Compt Rend de Soc de Biol* 1891; seance 19 December; 3:841–2.

39. Gley E. Experimentelle Untersuchungen über die Bedeutung der Schilddrüse und ihren Nebendrüsen für den Organismus. *Pflügers Archiv* 1897; 66 (No. 5–6): 308–19.

Gley E. Bemerkungen über die Funktion der Schilddrüse und ihrer Nebendrüsen. *Plügers Arch* 1896; 66:308–19.

Gley E. The pathogeny of exophthalmic goitre. *BMJ* 1901; 21 September:771–3.

Vassale G, Generali F. Fonction parathyroidienne et fonction thyroidienne. *Arch Ital Biol* 1896; 33:154–5.

Vassale G, Generali F. On the effects of exstirpation of the parathyroid glands. *Alien & Neurol* 1897; 18:57–61.

40. *The Nobel Archives*. Nobel Forum. Evaluation of G Vassale: C Sundberg (1905).

Bliss M. *The Discovery of Insulin*. Toronto: University of Toronto Press, 3rd ed. 2000.

41. Comroe JH. Missed opportunities. *Am Rev Respir Dis* 1976; 114:1167–73.

Meyers MA. *Happy Accidents. Serendipity in Modern Medical Breakthroughs*. New York: Arcade Publ. 2007.

MacCallum WG, Welch WH. *William Stewart Halsted, Surgeon*. Baltimore: The Johns Hopkins Press, 1930.

43. Pineles F. Klinische und experimentelle Beiträge zur Physiologie der Schilddrüse und der Epithelkörperchen. *Mitteil aus d Grenzgebiet der Med und Chir* 1905; Band 14:120.

5. The calcium connection

p.44. Ringer S. A further contribution regarding the influence of the different constituents of the blood on the contraction of the heart. *J Physiol* 1883; 429–42.

Miller DJ. Sidney Ringer; physiological saline, calcium and the contraction of the heart. *J Physiol* 2004; 555.3:585–7.

46. Loeb J. On an apparently new form of muscular irritability (contact irritability?) produced by solutions of salts (preferentially sodium salts) whose anions are liable to form insoluble calcium compounds. *Am J Physiol* 1901; 5:362–73.

Loeb J. The role of salts in the preservation of life. *Science* 1911; 17 November: 653–65.

47. Pauly PJ. The invention of artificial parthenogenesis. In: *Contolling Life: Jacques Loeb and the Engineering Ideal in Biology*. New York: Oxford Univ Press, 1987, p. 93–117.

Boston Herald. The creation of life. 26 November, 1899.

Lewis S. *Arrowsmith*. New York: Signet Classic, 1998.

49. Sawin CT. What causes tetany after removal of the parathyroid glands? MacCallum, Voegtlin and calcium. *Endocrinologist* 2003; 13:1–3.

Jaiwal JK. Calcium – how and why? *J Biosci* 2001; 26:357–63.

Williams RJP. The evolution of calcium biochemistry. *Biochim Biophys Acta* 2006; 1763:1139–46.

Roland CG. Maude Abbott and J.B. MacCallum. Canadian cardiac pioneers. *Chest* 1970; 57:371–77.

MacCallum WG, Voegtlin C. On the relation of the parathyroid to calcium metabolism and the nature of tetany. *Bull Johns Hopkins Hosp* 1908; 19:91.

MacCallum WG, Voegtlin. On the relation of tetany to the parathyroid glands and to calcium metabolism. *J Exp Med* 1909; 11:118–51.

50. Parhon G, Ureche CS. *Revista Stiintelor Medicale* 1907; July-August.

Koch WF. On the occurence of methyl guanidine in the urine of parathyroidectomized animals. *J Biol Chem* 1912; 12:313–5.

51. MacCallum WG, Lambert RA, Vogel KM. The removal of calcium from the blood by dialysis in the study of tetany. *J Exp Med* 1914; 20:149–68.

Salvesen HA. Studies on the physiology of the parathyroids. *Acta Med Scand* 1923; Suppl. No. 6:1–159.

Mayor RH, Orr TG, Weber CJ. Observations on the blood guanidine in tetania parathyreopriva. *Bull Johns Hopkins Hosp* 1927; 40:287–96.

Dolev E. A Gland in search of a function: the parathyroid glands and the explanations of tetany 1903–1926. *J Hist Med Allied Sci* 1987; 42:186–98.

52. Berridge MJ. Calcium signalling, a spatiotemporal phenomen. In: J Krebs and M Michalak (eds), *New Comprehensive Biochemistry*. Elsevier, 2007, vol.41: 485–502.

53. Okabe M, Graham A. The origin of the parathyroid gland. *PNAS* 2004; 101:17716–9.

Chang W, Shoback D. Extracellular Ca2+ -sensing receptors – an overview. *Cell Calcium* 2004; 35:183–96.

54. Miller S. Calcitonin – guardian of the mammalian skeleton or is it just a fish story? *Endocrinology* 2006; 147:4007–9.

Woodrow JP, Sharpe CJ, *et al.* Calcitonin plays a critical role in regulating skeletal mineral metabolism during lactation. *Endocrinology* 2006; 147:4010–21.

55. Stokes GG. The change in the refrangibility of light or fluorescence. *Royal Soc Archives* 1852. London: Royal Society.

Tsien RY. Unlocking cell secrets with light beams and molecular spies. *Heineken Lectures* 2002. www.knaw.nl

Grynkiewicz G, Poenie M, *et al.* A new generation of Ca2+ indicators with greatly improved fluorescence properties. *J Biol Chem* 1985; 260:3440–50.

56. Mithal A, Brown EM. An overview of extracellular homeostasis and the roles of the CaR in parathyroid and C-cells. In: Chattopadhyay N, Brown EM (eds): *Calcium-sensing receptors.* Boston: Kluwer Academic Publ, 2003, p. 1–27.

6. Hormones and organotherapy

p.58. Starling EH. Croonian Lecture: On the chemical correlation of the functions of the body I. *Lancet* 1905; 2:339–341.

59. Lewis S. *Arrowsmith.* New York: Signet Classic, 1998.

Murray GR. Note on the treatment of myxedema by hypodermic injections of the thyroid gland of a sheep. *BMJ* 1891; 2:796–7.

Moussu G. Sur la fonction parathyroidienne. *Comp de Rend Soc de Biol* 1898; 50:867–69.

Easterbrook CC. The action of thyroid and parathyroid extracts upon metabolism in the insane. *Lancet* 1898; Vol. 2, 27 August:546–549.

61. Réal J. *Voronoff.* Eugene, Oregon: Stock Publ., 2001.

Bulgakov M. *The Heart of a Dog.* London: Vintage, Random House, 2005.

63. Cushing H. Disorders of the pituitary gland. Retrospective and prophetic. *JAMA* 1921; 3:253–61.

Bliss M. *Harvey Cushing. A life in Surgery.* New York: Oxford University Press, 2005.

64. Rowntree LG. An evaluation of therapy with special reference to organotherapy. *Endocrinology* 1925; 9:1181–91.

7. The priority dispute

p.66. Li A. JB Collip, AM Hanson and the isolation of the parathyroid hormone, or endocrines and enterprise. *J Hist Med All Sci* 1992; 47:405–38.

Hanson AM. An elementary chemical study of the parathyroid glands of cattle. *Military Surg* 1923; March: 1–5.

Carney JA. The glandulae parathyroidea of Ivar Sandström. Contributions from two continents. *Am J Surg Path* 1996; 20:1123–44.

Hanson AM. A brief history of the family of Adolph Melanchton Hanson and Marie Martin Hanson as recorded by their son. March 1989. AM Hanson papers. Owen Wangensteen Historical Library, University of Minnesota.

68. Schein M. Aphorisms & quotations for the surgeon. Shewsbury, UK: Tfm Publ, 2003, p.143.

69. Cushing H. Letter to A. M. Hanson. 24 June, 1924; AM Hanson papers. Owen Wangensteen Historical Library, University of Minnesota.

71. Bliss M. Resurrections in Toronto: the emergence of insulin. *Horm Res* 2005; 64 (Suppl. 2): 98–102.

Bliss M. *The Discovery of Insulin*. Chicago: University of Chicago Press, 1982.

Rosenfeld L. Insulin: discovery and controversy. *Clin Chem* 2002; 48:2270–88.

Collip JB. Frederick Grant Banting, discoverer of insulin. *Sci Monthly* 1941; 52:473–4.

73. Collip JB, Leitch DB. A case of tetany treated with Parathyrin. *CMAJ* 1925; 15:59–60.

Li A. *JB Collip and the Development of Medical Research in Canada. Extracts and Enterprise*. Montreal: McGill-Queen's University Press, 2003.

74. Cushing H. Letter to A. M. Hanson. 11 April, 1925. AM Hanson papers. Owen Wangensteen Historical Library, University of Minnesota.

75. Hanson AM. Letter to H. Cushing. 15 April, 1925. AM Hanson papers. Owen Wangensteen Historical Library, University of Minnesota.

76. Hanson AM. Experiments with active preparations of parathyroid other than that of desiccated gland. *Military Surgeon* 1924; 53:701–18.

Cushing H. Letter to A. M. Hanson. 25 February 1924. *AM Hanson papers*. Owen Wangensteen Historical Library, University of Minnesota.

78. *The Saint Paul Pioneer Press*. Doctor given Gold Medal for Gland Discovery. 24 May, 1933.

The Nobel Archives. Nobel Forum. Evaluation of JB Collip: Liljestrand G (1928); Hammarsten E (1936); von Euler U (1944); Hammarsten E (1951).

79. Munson PL. Parathyroid hormone and calcitonin. In: *Endocrinology: People and Ideas*. McCann SM (ed.). Bethesda: American Physiological Society, 1988. p. 265–68.

8. Immortal patients

p.81. Sims WS. *The Victory at Sea*. London: John Murray, 1921.

Evening Express, Liverpool, 11 April, 1917. US Armed Ship. The New York mined near Mersey.

The Daily Mail. 11 April, 1917. US liner mined. Mishap 35 miles from Liverpool.

84. Albright F. A page out of the history of hyperparathyroidism. *J Clin Endocrinol* 1948; 8:637–57.

Bauer W, Federman DD. Hyperparathyroidism epitomized: the case of Captain Charles E. Martell. *Metabolism* 1962; 11:21–29.

Niederle BE, Schmidt G, *et al*. Albert J and his surgeon: a historical reevaluation of the first parathyroidectomy. *J Am Coll Surg* 2006; 202:181–90.

85. Mandl F. Therapeutischer Versuch bei Osteitis fibrosa generalisata mittels Exstirpation eines Epithelkörpsrchentumors. *Wien Klin Wochenschr* 1925; 50:1343–4.

Mandl F. Therapeutischer Versuch bei einem Falle von Osteitis fibrosa generalisata mittels Exstirpation eines Epithelkörperschentumors. *Zentralbl f Chirurgie* 1926; 5:260–64.

Mandl F. Klinisches und Experimentelles zur Frage der lokalisierten und generalisierten Osteitis fibrosa. *Arch f Chir* 1926; 143:245–84.

86. Gold E. Über die bedeutung der epithelkörperchenvergrössung bei der Osteitis fibrosa generalisata Recklinghausen. *Mitt Grenzgeb Med Chir* 1927; 41:63–82.

87. Roland CG. Hyperparathyroidism. Some early patients. *Arch. Intern Med* 1970; 126:558–566.

Spence HM. The life and death of Captain Charles Martell and kidney stone disease. *J Urol* 1984; 132:1204–7.

88. Hunter D, Aub JC. Lead studies. XV. The effect of the parathyroid hormone on the excretion of lead and calcium in patients suffering from lead poisoning. *Quart J Med* 1927; January: 123–4.

89. Montagne P. No. 53 – History of precaution. *Rachel's Environment & Health News*, 26 March, 1997.

Bryson B. *A Short History of Nearly Everything.* London: Black Swan, 2004, pp. 193–205.

Means JH. Ward 4. The Mallinckrodt Research Ward of the Massachusetts General Hospital. In: In honor of Fuller Albright: father of modern endocrinology. Kolb F (ed.). *The Endocrinologist* 2000; Suppl:90–100.

90. Axelrod L. Bones, stones and hormones: the contributions of Fuller Albright. *N Engl J Med* 1970; 283:964–70.

Personal communication: Rolf Luft, 2006.

92. Cope O. The story of hyperparathyroidism at the Massachusetts General Hospital. In: In honor of Fuller Albright: father of modern endocrinology. Kolb F (ed.). *The Endocrinologist* 2000; suppl:101–2.

Bergstrand H. Osteitis fibrosa generalisata Recklinghausen mit pluriglandulärer Affektion der innersekretorischen Drüsen und röntgenologisch nachweisbarem Parathyroideatumor. *Acta Med Scand* 1931; 76:128–52.

9. A disease in disguise

p.95. *Lancet* 1933; 2 September:547–8.

Albright F, *et al.* Studies on physiology of parathyroid glands. IV. *Am J Med Sci* 1934; 187:49–61.

96. Cope O, Barnes BA, *et al.* Vicissitudes of parathyroid surgery. Trials of diagnosis and management in 51 patients with a variety of disorders. *Ann Surg* 1961; 154:491–506.

98. WT St. Goar coined the phrase: "bones, stones and abdominal groans". *Ann Intern Med* 1957; 46:102.

Randall RV, Keating FR. The serendipity in diagnosis of primary hyperparathyroidism. *Am J Med Sci* 1958; 236:575–89.

The Three Princes of Serendip http://livingheritage.org/three_princes.htm

99. Haff RC, Black WC, Ballinger WF. Primary hyperparathyroidism: changing clinical, surgical and pathological aspects. *Ann Surg* 1970; 171:85–92.

Boonstra CE, Jackson CE. Hyperparathyroidism detected by routine serum calcium analysis. *Ann Intern Med* 1965; 63:468–74.

Wermers RA, Khosla S, et al. The rise and fall of primary hyperparathyroidism: a population-based study in Rochester, Minnesota, 1965–1992. *Ann Intern Med* 1997; 126:433–40.

Lundgren E, et al. Population-based screening for primary hyperparathyroidism with serum calcium and parathyroid hormone values in menopausal women. *Surgery* 1997; 121:287–94.

100. Illich I. *Limits to Medicine. Medical Nemesis: The Expropriation of Health.* London: Marion Boyars Publ, 3rd ed. 2002.

Hadler NM. *The Last Well Person: How to Stay Well Despite the Health-Care System.* Montreal: McGill-Queen's University Press, 2004.

101. Norman G. The epistemology of clinical reasoning: perspectives from philosophy, psychology and neuroscience. *Acad Med* 2000; 75:S127–33.

Campbell EJM, et al. The concept of disease. *BMJ* 1979; 2:757–62.

Smith R. In search of "non-disease". *BMJ* 2002; 324:883–5.

102. Consensus Development Conference Panel. Diagnosis and management of asymptomatic primary hyperparathyroidism: Consensus development conference statement. *Ann Intern Med* 1991; 114:593–97.

103. Nordenström J, Strigård KJ, et al. Hyperparathyroidism associated with treatment of manic-depressive disorders by lithium. *Eur J Surg* 1992; 158:207–11.

Cade J. Lithium salt in the treatment of psychotic excitement. *Med J Aus* 1949; 3 September: 349–51.

10. The elusive hormone

p.105. Collip JB. The extraction of a parathyroid hormone which will prevent or control parathyroid tetany and which regulates the level of blood calcium. *J Biol Chem* 1925; 63:395–438.

Potts JT. Parathyroid hormone: past and present. *J Endocrinol* 2005; 187:311–25.

Gladwell M. Open secrets. *The New Yorker*, 8 January, 2007; 44–53.

106. Auerbach GD. Isolation of parathyroid hormone after extraction with phenol. *J Biol Chem* 1959; 12:3179–81.

Brewer HB, Ronan R. Bovine parathyroid hormone: amino acid sequence. *Proc Nat Acad Sci* 1970; 67:1862–9.

D'Amour P. Circulating PTH molecular forms: what we know and what we don't. *Kidney Int* 2006; 70:529–33.

107. Yalow R, Berson SA. Immunoassay of endogenous plasma insulin. *J Clin Invest* 1960; 39:1157–75.

Yalow R. Radioimmunoassay: a probe for the study for the fine structure of biological systems. *Science* 1978; 200:1236–45.

109. Straus E. *Rosalyn Yalow. Nobel Laureate. Her Life and Work in Medicine.* New York: Plenum Trade, 1998.

110. Rall JE, Berson SA. Biographical memoirs. Washington D.C., *National Acad Sci* 1990:55–62.

Berson SA, Yalow RS, *et al.* Immunoassay of bovine and human parathyroid hormone. *Proc Nat Acad Sci* 1963; 49:613–7.

112. Silverman R, Yalow RS. Heterogeneity of parathyroid hormone. Clinical and physiological implications. *J Clin Invest* 1973; 52:1958–71.

113. Doppman JL. Reoperative parathyroid surgery: localization procedures. *Prog Surg* 1986; 18:117–32.

Coakley AJ, Kettle AG, *et al.* 99-Tc-m sestamibi – a new agent for parathyroid imaging. *Nucl Med Commun* 1989; 10:791–4.

Morgenstein L. The decline and fall of the surgical incision. *Surg Innov* 2006; 13:207–8.

114. Litynski GS. Erich Mühe and the rejection of cholecystectomy (1985): a surgeon ahead of his time. *JSLS* 1998; 2:341–6.

11. The language of god

p.116. Mendel G. Versuche über Pflanzen-Hybriden. Transact af Verhandlungen des naturforschenden Vereines in Brünn (1865). 1866; iv:3–270. Reprinted in: *BMJ* 1965; i:367–74.

Jay V. Gregor Johann Mendel. *Arch Pathol Lab Med* 2001; 125:320–1.

117. Brown EM.The pathophysiology of primary hyperparathyroidism. *J Bone Mineral Res* 2002; Suppl.2:N24–9.

Brown EM, Gamba G, *et al.* Cloning and characterization of an extracellular Ca– 2+ – sensing receptor from bovine parathyroid. *Nature* 1993; 366:575–80.

119. Potts JT, Gardella TJ, *et al.* The history of parathyroid hormone and its receptor: structure-based design of parathyroid hormone analogues. *Osteoporos Int* 1997; 7 (Suppl. 3): S169–73.

Gensure RG, Gardella TJ, *et al.* Parathyroid hormone-related peptide, and their receptors. *Biochem Biophys Res Commun* 2004; 328:666–78.

120. Nemeth EF, Fox J. Calcimimetic compounds: a direct approach to controlling plasma levels of parathyroid hormone in hyperparathyroidism. *Trends Endocrinol Metab* 1999; 10:66–71.

Wüthrich RP, Martin D, Bilezikian JP. The role of calcimetics in the treatment of hyperparathyroidism. *Eur J Clin Invest* 2007; 37:915–22.

121. Gawande A. The way we age now. *The New Yorker*, 30 April, 2007.

122. Arnold A, Shattuck TM, *et al.* Molecular pathogenesis of primary hyperparathyroidism. *J Bone Mineral Res* 2002; 17 (suppl. 2): N30–6.

123. Knudson A. Mutation and cancer: statistical study of retinoblastoma. *Proc Natl Acad Sci* 1971; 68:820–3.

    Jackson CE. The two-hit theory of neoplasia: implications for the pathogenesis of hyperparathyroidism. *Cancer Genetics and Cytogenetics* 1985; 14:175–8.

    Whitaker Hulke J. Pathological Society of London report. *BMJ* 1884; 5 April:687–8.

124. Erdheim J. Zur normalen und Patologischen histologie der glandula thyroidea, parathyroidea und hypophysis. *Beitr z Path Anath* 1903; 33:158–236.

12. The pharmacological paradox

p.126. Johnell O, Kanis JA. An estimate of the worldwide prevalence, mortality and disability associated with hip fracture. *Osteoporos Int* 2004; 15:897–902.

127. Bauer W, Aud JC, Albright F. Studies of calcium and phosphorus metabolism V. *J Exp Med* 1929; 49:145–62.

    Albright F, *et al.* Studies of calcium and phosphorus metabolism IV. The effect of the parathyroid hormone. *JCI* 1929; 7:139–81.

    Rosch PJ. Reminiscences of Hans Selye, and the birth of "stress." *Health and Stress* 1997; 9:1–8.

    Pugsley LI, Selye H. The histological changes in the bone responsible for the action of parathyroid hormone on the calcium metabolism of the rat. *J Physiol* 1933; 79:113–7.

128. Le Fanu J. *The Rise and Fall of Modern Medicine.* London: Abacus, 2000, p.22.134. The Nobel Archives, Nobel Forum. Evaluation of H Selye: U von Euler (1955 och 1949).

129. Jubiz W, Canterbury JM, Tyler FH. Circadian rhythm in serum Parathyroid hormone concentration in human subjects: correlation with serum calcium, phosphate, albumin and growth hormone levels. *J Clin Invest* 1972; 51:2040–6.

    Markowitz ME, Arnaud S, *et al.* Temporal interrelationships between the circadian rhythms of serum parathyroid hormone and calcium concentrations. *JCEM* 1988; 67:1068–73.

    Lobaugh B, Neelon FA, *et al.* Circadian rhythms for calcium, inorganic phosphorus and parathyroid hormone in primary hyperparathyroidism: functional and practical implications. *Surgery* 1989; 106:1009–17.

130. Schibler U. Circadian time keeping: the daily ups and downs of genes, cells and organismus. *Prog Brain Res* 2006; 153:271–82.

    Ohdo S. Chronopharmacology focused on biological clock. *Drug Metab Pharmacokinet* 2007; 22:3–14.

Martin TJ, Quinn JMT *et al*. Mechanisms involved in skeletal anabolic thera-pies. *Ann N Y Acad Sci* 2006; 1068:458–70.

Shoback D. Update in osteoporosis and metabolic bone disorders. *JCEM* 2007; 92:747–53.

Cranney A, Papaioannou A, *et al*. Parathyroid hormone for the treatment of osteoporosis: a systematic review. *CMAJ* 2006; 175:52–9.

Neer RM, Arnaud CD, *et al*. Effect of parathyroid hormone (1–34) on frac-tures and bone mineral density in postmenopausal women with osteo-porosis. *N Eng J Med* 2001; 344:1434–41.

Aspenberg P, Genant HK *et al*. Teriparatide for acceleration of fracture repair in humans: a prospective, randomized, double-blind study of 102 post-menopausal women with distal radial fractures. *J Bone Miner Res* 2010; 25:404–14.

131. Albright F, Reifenstein EC. *The Parathyroid Glands and Metabolic Bone Disease*. Baltimore: Williams and Wilkins, 1948.

Carroll L. *The Hunting of the Snark*. London: Macmillan, 1876.

Index

The Hunt for the Parathyroids, First Edition. Jörgen Nordenström.
© 2013 John Wiley & Sons, Ltd. Published 2013 by John Wiley & Sons, Ltd.

██████████

Printed and bound by CPI Group (UK) Ltd, Croydon, CR0 4YY

Printed and bound by CPI Group (UK) Ltd, Croydon, CR0 4YY

27/10/2024

14580211-0001